EXTRA LOVE: THE ART OF HANDS-ON ASSISTS
THE DEFINITIVE MANUAL FOR YOGA TEACHERS, ASSISTANTS AND ADVANCED STUDENTS

VOLUME TWO: STANDING POSES, BACK BENDS & SURYA NAMASKAR

BY JILL ABELSON, 500 ERYT, ADVANCED CERTIFIED JIVAMUKTI YOGA TEACHER

Extra Love: The Art of Hands-On Assists
The Definitive Manual for Yoga Teachers, Assistants and Advanced Students
Volume Two: Standing Poses, Back Bends & Surya Namaskar

Copyright © Jill Abelson 2012

ISBN: 978-0-615-70840-9

Printed and bound in the USA

Cover Design, Design, Typesetting & Print Production
by Michael Fantasia
www.linkedin.com/in/mfantasia

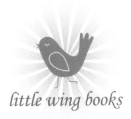

Little Wing Books
San Francisco, California

Jill Abelson
www.yogaofliberation.com
San Francisco, CA 94114

Cover Illustration "The Nadis, diagram, Tibet"

TABLE OF CONTENTS

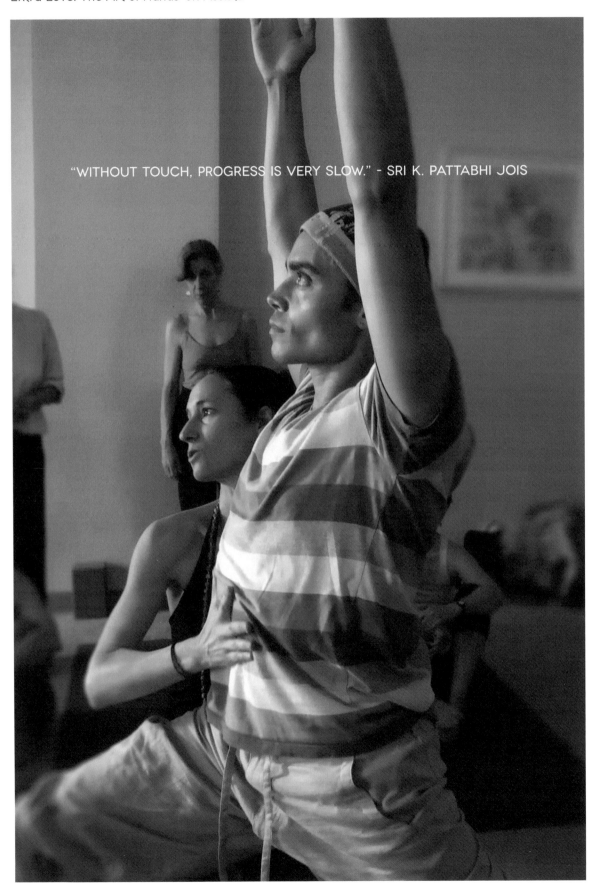

"WITHOUT TOUCH, PROGRESS IS VERY SLOW." - SRI K. PATTABHI JOIS

INTRODUCTION

In the twelve months since publishing *EXTRA LOVE: The Art of Hands-on-Assists, Volume One: Hips, Twists & Forward Bends*, I've heard from teachers all over the country with enthusiastic praise about the book. Teachers have unanimously appreciated its simplicity, clarity, technical precision and overall value as a teaching resource. Many teachers said they were able to put the information to use right away, benefitting from the book's immediate application in the classroom. I wanted the book to be practical and was thrilled to get so much positive feedback. With this wave of encouragement, I sat down to tackle Volume 2, covering Standing Poses, Back Bends & Surya Namaskar.

"Why give hands-on adjustments?" A new teacher asked this question at a recent workshop in San Francisco. My answer: to prevent injury, ensure safety and encourage proper alignment; to help remove or overcome physical, emotional, energetic or other blockages students may experience during class; to provide reassuring support; to take students deeper in poses than they may have ever gone. You might say that assists help students "cross over" to the other side. Plus, it simply feels great to receive and to give, erasing the physical barrier between student and teacher, deepening the relationship for both parties.

Like the first volume, this second manual condenses more than thirteen years of teaching and assisting every kind of student imaginable: all ages, shapes and sizes. In six years of offering my assisting workshops and trainings, I've found that many teachers would like to assist more, but don't yet have the confidence or skills—increasingly important as yoga and teacher training programs grow in popularity and new generations of teachers are called to serve their communities. I've met 200-hour teacher training program graduates who never had the opportunity to touch a student during their entire training. Teachers with a knack for assisting come to my workshops several times and take away a little bit more each time. The book includes insights and examples from my travels far and wide teaching the material and leading and assisting very large group classes. This ongoing experience gives me a level of assisting expertise that I have not yet found in other books or technical resources and which I joyfully share with you.

"A PERSON REACHES ENLIGHTENMENT 75% MORE QUICKLY WITH HANDS-ON ASSISTS." – DAVID LIFE

WHAT YOU WILL GET FROM THIS MANUAL

This manual is organized just like my workshops. You will first read about general principles of assisting, followed by organized, detailed recommendations and tips for Standing Poses, Back Bends and Surya Namaskar.[1]

Following the format of the first book, I include common misalignments to look for, as well as recommended assists for each pose. I aimed to write the text clearly enough so that as you read along, you will have a good idea of what to look for, as well as how to assist the poses covered. I also include options for assisting beginning, intermediate, advanced and all-levels students.

In selecting among many poses, I've chosen several all-time-greatest-hits that are popular in today's classes, well known and accessible to students of all levels. Thumbnail photos will enhance your understanding of the text. There is a short, must-read section on **Ethics/Safety**, as well as a **Resources** section at the end to help you find related material and skills. Additional and advanced poses—including Inversions—will be covered in the next volume of this series.

Pep talk: I always advise teachers to start small and develop their inventory of skills first. Owing to the almost complete lack of touch in our daily lives, putting your hands on students—and feeling their receptivity in return—can be an intimidating experience. To assist well means, in essence, mastering the art of nonverbal communication: you're able to read the body and respond effectively. For Surya Namaskar, you also need a good sense of timing and rhythm.

Soon you will sharpen your eye and develop a sixth sense about why and how to give an amazing assist to any type of student in any pose. Though there are infinite permutations in physical bodies and the possible expression of the poses, you'll start to notice common threads and be able to apply assisting principles from one pose to another. You'll get better at understanding what to look for, easily identify common misalignments and know what to do. I strongly believe in the value of assisting your own teachers in their classes, where you're not responsible for the entire class, yet are contributing to individual students and their depth of experience.

"INTUITION IS NOT A GIFT BUT A SKILL." - CAROLYN MYSS

For a deeper dive into this special material, please seek out my workshops, which focus on principals and techniques of assists, covering all categories of poses. As in the book, I teach how to assist with confidence from a technical standpoint, as well as what to look for—and why—in order to optimize students' alignment and energy flow, ensure their safety and deepen their experience and joy of Yoga. We discuss student and teacher comfort, injury prevention and ethical considerations. You have the opportunity to practice hands-on assists throughout the entire workshop. It is an ideal course for new and experienced teachers, teaching assistants and advanced students wishing to deepen their knowledge and strengthen their connection with students.

This manual is an offering to the incomparable master teachers who gave me love for the "extra love": my primary teachers Sharon Gannon and David Life, founders of Jivamukti Yoga; Yoganand Michael Carroll of Kripalu Yoga; David Swenson, master teacher of Ashtanga Vinyasa Yoga; Lucy Bowen-McCauley, dance educator and choreographer; and Dody DiSanto, performer, movement instructor, body worker and dear friend.

---

1 *EXTRA LOVE: The Art of Hands on Assists Volume One: Hips, Twists & Forward Bends* was originally prepared to accompany my workshops at the Yoga Alliance National Leadership Conference in 2011.

PRINCIPLES OF ASSISTING

Concentrate – Your full concentration is needed when assisting students. It sounds straightforward, but it's challenging to assist one or multiple students, while simultaneously instructing a group, calling out poses, maintaining the rhythm of a class, tending to your music playlist, etc. Place your full concentration on the student being assisted, while keeping your antenna up toward the rest of class. Figure that if teaching class requires 100 percent of your attention and focus, assisting students will require 200 percent!

Have an Intention – A great assist always starts with a road map. It's important to know technically what you are going for in an assist and why. This means looking at a student, drawing on your own knowledge/understanding of the pose inside and out, knowing how the pose functions and knowing how to optimize alignment. I would also point out that it is helpful to approach assists as enhancements rather than "fixes." Start where the student is and go from there. I once heard a new teacher say (referring to a student), "He couldn't even do Down Dog!!" which suggested to me the teacher was probably stomping around the classroom, grumpily fixing what he saw as "wrong." Not exactly an ideal attitude. Knowledge, skill and insight come with time and a little patience.

Use Breath – Proper breathing is the cornerstone of Yoga practice – it directly increases strength, stretch, endurance and balance and gets students into their bodies. Pay attention to students' breath. Familiarize yourself with the basic anatomy of breathing, how the breath travels in the body. Train your ears to listen for and eyes to watch the breath. Use audible *ujjayi* when assisting. With experience, you will be able to see where the breath might be getting stuck in the body and how to facilitate its movement and flow.

MANY TEACHERS WORK FROM THE TOP (OR PERIPHERY) DOWN - WHICH ADDRESSES THE EDGES OF A POSE, WHILE MISSING THE FOUNDATION. A STUDENT NEEDS A SOLID FOUNDATION TO PROGRESS AND TO FEEL CONNECTED ON MANY LEVELS.

Know Energy – Since Yoga is meant to facilitate the flow of energy and prana in the body, it's important to know HOW energy moves. Knowledge of Yoga anatomy and the subtle body (chakras, nadis, bandhas) is very helpful. Know the lines of energy for the various poses and be able to help students direct energy to parts of the body through hands-on and verbal assists. Many Yoga classes focus on the outer, muscular form of the body. I'm suggesting here that you tune into the subtle, inner body and help students understand poses from the inside out. Several outstanding books on Yoga anatomy/alignment are listed under Resources.

Earth First! – I'm fortunate to come from a lineage – Jivamukti Yoga – that interprets asana (or pose) as a steady, joyful connection to the **earth**. An effective assist helps to reassert that connection for a student, grounding them back to home base. The connection to the earth will be through the student's hands, feet, seat, head – whatever is in contact with the ground. When assisting, it is good to train your eyes to look at the base first, then work your way up. For example, in standing poses, you would first address foot pattern/placement and placement of feet relative to hips/rest of body. A steady seat is required for seated poses, hip openers and twists. Many teachers work from the top (or periphery) down — which addresses the edges of a pose, while missing the foundation. A student needs a solid foundation to progress and to feel connected, on many levels.

Prioritize — If you are new to hands-on assisting, the hardest part is prioritizing — knowing which assists to do first, then being able to rank order what to do next according to individual or group needs. This is not really a matter of personal preference so much as safety. I typically address students with major misalignments and/or potential for injury FIRST, followed by foundation issues (connection to the earth), minor misalignments, stress/fear response, then other enhancements to outer form and then fine tuning for the inner body. Practice being able to quickly diagnose what's happening collectively and individually, as you offer enhancements and support.

Honor Pain — Teachers often ask me, "When assisting, how do you know how far to go?" This insight comes from direct experience, getting to know your students' bodies, their normal range of flexibility and strength and typical resistance points in a pose.

Be receptive to any pain, injuries or physical limitations or blockages. Before class, you might ask new (or continuing) if students have any injuries. One studio I know of has students write down their injuries on index cards, to place on their mats before class. Drawing from your own experience and careful student observation, you will learn to recognize resistance points in the body and tailor your assists accordingly. To that I would add: learn to tell the difference between pain (physical or psychological discomfort) and intensity (working at the edge but not risking injury). Tell-tale signs of pain and discomfort are changes in breath, changes in skin tone/color, bulging or tense expression of eyes, white knuckles, or changes in facial expression. Intense grimacing is not a good sign. If you see this in *your* class, go over and support that student ASAP, or take it as a cue that the class as a whole may benefit from slowing down, focusing on breaking down the pose, or taking a rest in Child's Pose.

YOUR JOB IS TO KEEP EVERYONE SAFE WITHIN THEIR OWN ABILITIES. A NONCOMPETITIVE/NON-JUDGMENTAL MOOD WILL REFLECT IN THE GENEROSITYOF YOUR ASSISTS ACROSS A BROAD SPECTRUM OF STUDENTS AND LEVELSOF PROFICIENCY.

Set Mood — Before class begins, I often ask students to say hi to the people sitting nearby and maybe share something great about their day. It's a nice way to warm up the room and above all establish a democratic feeling, as in "We're all in this together." Yoga is presented as non-competitive, but that doesn't mean it's free from competition. A student might compete against herself, driving toward an unreasonable goal, or against what appears to be the "average" level of the class judging from students around her. Your job is to keep everyone safe within their own abilities, helping students accept responsibility for their own bodies.

A non-competitive/non-judgmental mood will reflect in the generosity of your assists across a broad spectrum of students and levels of proficiency. Easier though it may be to assist competent, advanced students, you do so at the risk of alienating or endangering new or continuing students whose developing practice calls for more of your attention and care. Finally, it's completely appropriate to ask permission before assisting any student, or to announce before class your use of hands-on adjustments, should some students prefer to opt out for any reason.

Individualize/Vary your Approach – As much as possible, strive to individualize and effectively vary your approach, offering something slightly different for each person. There is no one magic assist for each pose. Familiarize yourself with appropriate assists for beginners to advanced students, for various body types, for both genders. Knowledge of the *chakra* system (see under Energetics) and Ayurvedic body types – *kapha, pitta* or *vata* – is also very helpful. *Chakra* strengths and imbalances, as well as strong ayurvedic constitutions, will reveal themselves during class – you want to know how to address them effectively. Learn, practice and perfect more than one assist for every pose, so you have a wide vocabulary to draw upon for all students.

It's common for newer and even experienced teachers to feel fear, insecurity or even aversion to assisting some students and not others, or a fear of assisting challenging students. Use all these feelings to learn. You might offer to work separately with an individual student after class, saying, "I've never worked with someone like you before – can we work together for a few minutes? I have some ideas that might help you." That way, you build confidence with injuries, different students and body types. I always offer this for students with chronic lower back pain, hand or shoulder alignment that is preventing a safe Downward Facing Dog, hyper-extension, scoliosis, or other unique conditions.

Use Options – All of my teachers have encouraged me to use options and find ways to creatively solve problems when assisting. I consistently draw on my own knowledge of the poses and use that information to address students' needs. It is not – by any stretch – "one-size-fits-all." Therein lies the art behind doing this well. Keep in mind that repeating details, using different words or suggestions, will help you reach more students. Explain what is good in the pose, using positive reinforcement, as well as what you are doing and why, so students can "download" your guidance and apply it throughout their practice.

Kripalu Yoga teachers are trained to apply six different types of assists: (1) a verbal assist – cuing or direction around alignment, form or essence of a pose; (2) demonstration – modeling a pose based on verbal cues; (3) "press point" or very light touch – to encourage lifting, lengthening, extension, etc.; (4) a manual assist – with one or both hands; (5) no assist at all ("that's fine!"); and (6) a restorative assist or brief massage. These all work beautifully in different situations. Know and use options.

Take Responsibility – A student's experience at ALL levels is YOUR responsibility. Do not attempt an assist unless you have 100% confidence. Practice and perfection of assists takes time. Then, once you're more confident with your observation, evaluation and assisting skills, be proactive in pointing out areas that need extra attention. For example, hyper-extension in Downward Facing Dog – or lack of lower back awareness in Upward Facing Dog – may lead to chronic lower back pain and injury over time. Lack of shoulder awareness in Chaturanga may lead to shoulder or arm injury. Be straightforward and honest about what you see, then use lots of positive reinforcement to call out immediate progress. Protect yourself as well (proper breath, *bandhas*, technique, insurance, ethical guidelines). There is more discussion under **Ethics/Safety Considerations**.

Practice Patience – One of my students first came to class with very rounded back and shoulders that seemed atypical for her age. I didn't assist her right away. Instead, I gave her a few weeks to settle into her body before I started to encourage length in her upper back. After a few months, she told me she works as a radiology nurse at a busy San Francisco hospital and wears a lead apron all day! The physical stress of her day job explained her posture, which through patience and discipline she enhanced to a beautiful, elegant form. Give students time to learn and process gradually and don't judge a book by its cover. A student many need a few or several classes to get acclimated. Use patience and consistency.

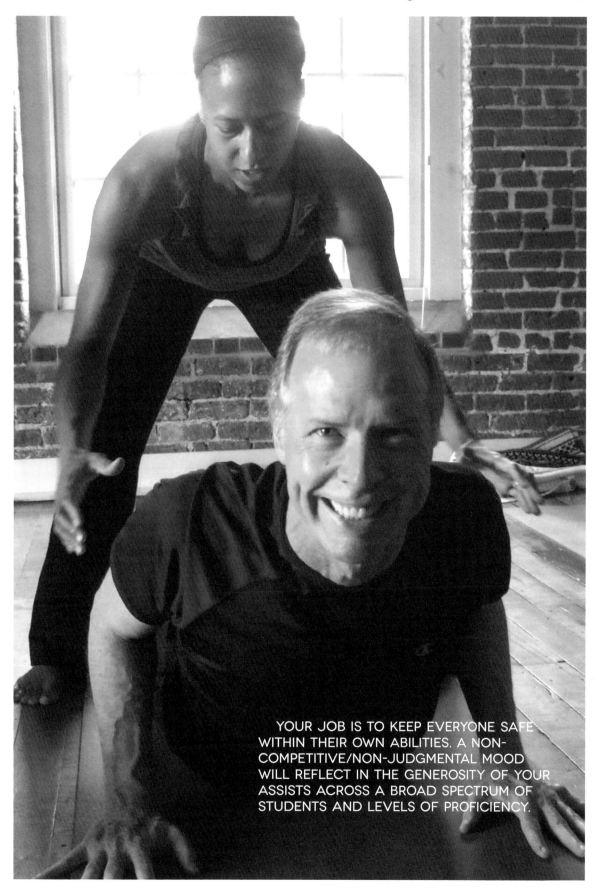

YOUR JOB IS TO KEEP EVERYONE SAFE WITHIN THEIR OWN ABILITIES. A NON-COMPETITIVE/NON-JUDGMENTAL MOOD WILL REFLECT IN THE GENEROSITY OF YOUR ASSISTS ACROSS A BROAD SPECTRUM OF STUDENTS AND LEVELS OF PROFICIENCY.

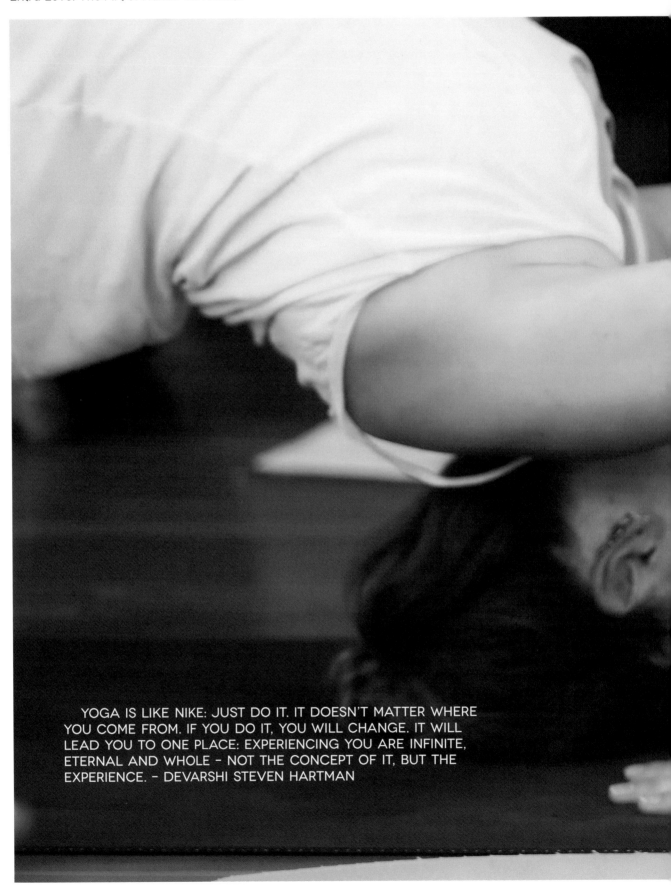

YOGA IS LIKE NIKE: JUST DO IT. IT DOESN'T MATTER WHERE YOU COME FROM. IF YOU DO IT, YOU WILL CHANGE. IT WILL LEAD YOU TO ONE PLACE: EXPERIENCING YOU ARE INFINITE, ETERNAL AND WHOLE - NOT THE CONCEPT OF IT, BUT THE EXPERIENCE. - DEVARSHI STEVEN HARTMAN

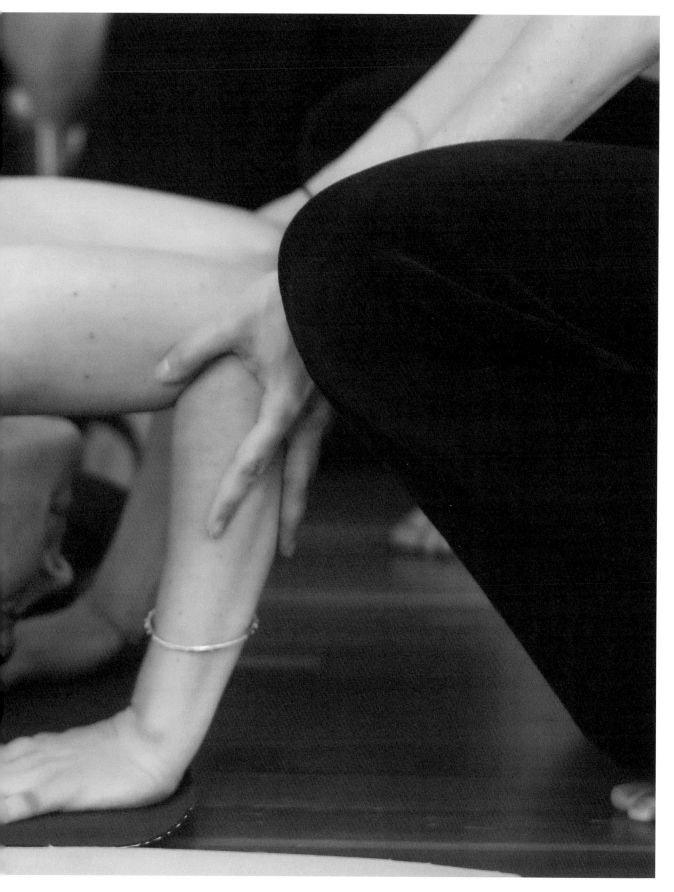

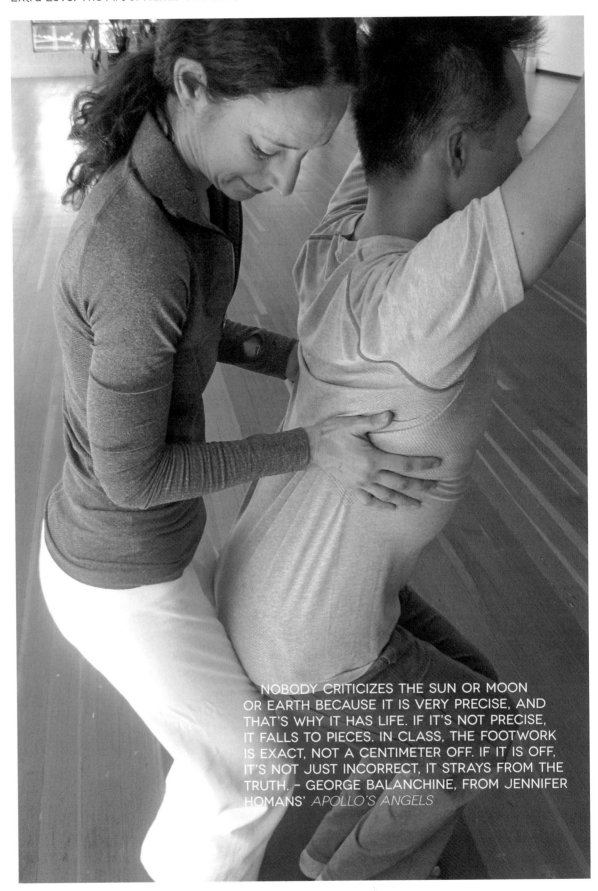

NOBODY CRITICIZES THE SUN OR MOON OR EARTH BECAUSE IT IS VERY PRECISE, AND THAT'S WHY IT HAS LIFE. IF IT'S NOT PRECISE, IT FALLS TO PIECES. IN CLASS, THE FOOTWORK IS EXACT, NOT A CENTIMETER OFF. IF IT IS OFF, IT'S NOT JUST INCORRECT, IT STRAYS FROM THE TRUTH. – GEORGE BALANCHINE, FROM JENNIFER HOMANS' *APOLLO'S ANGELS*

ASSISTING THE POSES

STANDING POSES

Standing poses are the building blocks of Hatha Yoga. They strengthen and bring mobility to the entire body. In teacher training, they're often the first poses we learn to teach, as well as the first poses accomplished by beginning students. My own teachers emphasize that standing poses represent our ability to be grounded, to stand on our own feet. Being grounded is essential to the attainment of Yoga—self-discovery, happiness and spiritual enlightenment.

In many *vinyasa* classes, standing poses make up the majority of the poses taught, with back bends, twists and inversions tucked in at the end. I used to put a lot of pressure on myself to stay on my feet the entire class. Eventually I got stronger and through both practicing and teaching, I began to closely observe the students around me. These experiences reinforced how small nuances and assists to standing poses can carry through our entire Yoga practice.

The first part of this section focuses on poses in which the hips are squared to the front. The second part looks at poses in which the hips are open to the side. For all the poses, foot pattern and even weight distribution are essential. Your objective is to stabilize the base first, then work from the ground up.

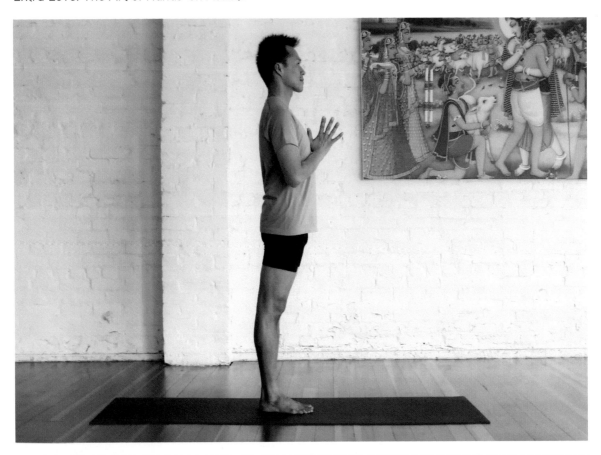

TADASANA—MOUNTAIN POSE

Tadasana—or *Samasthiti*—is the ultimate standing pose. *Tada* means mountain. *Sama* means upright, or straight. *Sthiti* means steady. The pose implies standing solid and tall as a mountain, steady at the base and conducting energy upward. *In Light on Yoga*, Master Iyengar reminds us that we often don't pay attention to our correct method of standing. Over time, uneven distribution of body weight leads to stiffness in the spine, strain and fatigue. Conscious placement of our weight, however, brings lightness, poise and balance to Tadasana and all standing poses. Our stance in Mountain Pose reflects how we see and carry ourselves in the world.

Teachers often assist Tadasana from the top, for example, rolling open the shoulders open, yet this type of assist addresses only the edges or periphery, while missing the foundation of the pose entirely. As you build confidence in assisting, you'll be able to diagnose and correct misalignments that will benefit your students' entire practices, giving them the greatest gift: learning how to stand on their own two feet, building body awareness, trust and inner confidence. In a natural landscape, everything is seen in relation to the mountain. So, too, in Yoga.

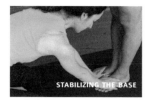
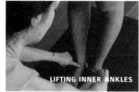
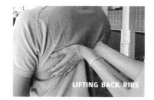
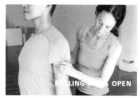

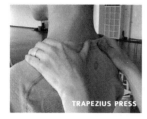
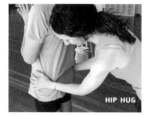
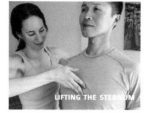
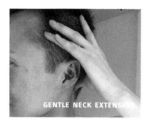

COMMON MISALIGNMENTS

- Uneven weight distribution on feet
- Feet turned in/out or not pressing into the floor—energy stuck in legs
- Knees hyper-extended

- Sagging in lower back or abdomen, slouching in upper back
- Head not balanced, chin forward or back

ASSISTS

Beginners: Stabilize the base first, working from bottom to top. Check for equal weight on feet. Have beginning students lift their toes and find equal weight distribution across all 4 corners of feet. Inner/outer balls of feet and inner/outer heels press down equally. Help student find steadiness by encouraging them to press feet firmly into the floor, then lifting energetically from the feet up through the shins, all the way UP the legs. Check to see that the feet aren't rolling in; if so, bring attention to inner ankles and suggest a "lifting up." Feet parallel, either together or hip-width apart.

If knees hyper-extend, suggest a small micro-bend or slight shift of weight forward on feet. A block squeezed sideways between the thighs helps activate the legs. Kneecaps lifted, quadriceps active.

Beginners/Intermediate: For a grounding assist, standing behind, hug and anchor the hips firmly *downward* with your hands to initiate a lifting up along the side body. This helps to anchor the pelvis over the legs. To adjust sagging in abdomen or lower back, stand to the side, placing one hand flat on sacrum, other hand flat on lower abdomen. Tailbone lengthens down without tucking, as lower abdomen lifts up. Side waists lengthen. Check to see that front ribs soften in. The torso is now aligned nicely over the pelvis. For lift through back body, gently hug and lift the back ribs. For the upper body, roll upper, inner arms open. Place your hands on the trapezius muscles as a reminder to release/soften the upper shoulders. Touch the sternum, to bring awareness and lift to upper chest.

Intermediate/Advanced: With a good foundation, you then have added options to refine the pose. Gently roll inner, upper arms open, rotating shoulders from the *sides*. Use a light touch/press point at the sternum and cue student to lift up against your touch. For length through neck and crown, put a hand (or block) flat on top of head and encourage student to lift up from feet through entire body (this is a fun assist to do with partners). Likewise, place your thumbs on the underside/occipital ridge of skull, with fingers lightly spread and placed around sides of head. Lift up *gently* to encourage extension. Finally, to release tension in the hands, sandwich the student's palm and help extend each hand parallel to side body, lengthening fingertips toward the ground. From these assists, you should see a nice lift through the upper body, with arms well aligned.

For Urdhva Hastasana (Tadasana with the arms overhead) many of these same assists apply. The hip hug is great to help anchor pelvis over legs and to prevent arching in lower back when arms lift overhead. Press trapezius muscles down and encourage inner, upper arms to open from the inside out: holding the biceps overhead, rotate upper arms so palms spin to face in toward center. Energy moves actively up the body as arms, hands and fingertips extend up. Side waists long, chest lifted with shoulders down. The pose should look alive!

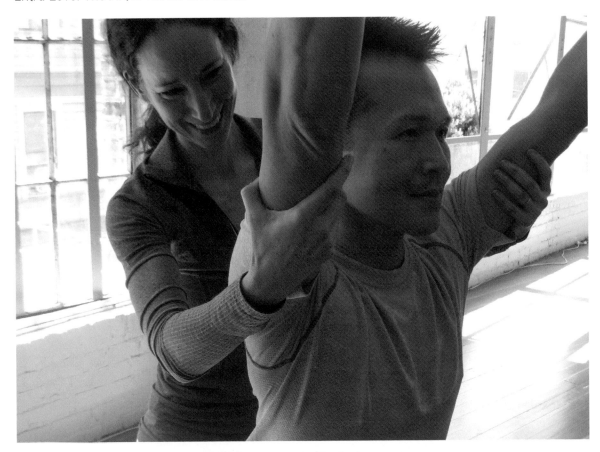

UTKATASANA—AWKWARD POSE

Utkatasana is a challenging standing pose, with the feet, knees and hips all establishing a square and even base. The feet and palms are either together or parallel. The legs are normally strong in this pose, but as the knees bend and pose is held, students may lose awareness of the lower back or upper body. Your approach to assisting here is similar to Mountain and Eagle Pose. Build a strong foundation, then work your way up.

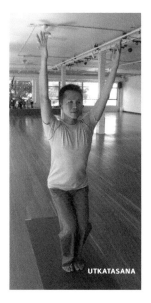
UTKATASANA

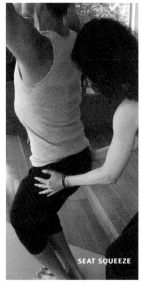
SEAT SQUEEZE

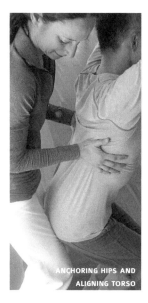
ANCHORING HIPS AND
ALIGNING TORSO

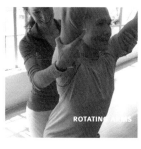
ROTATING ARMS

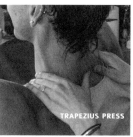
TRAPEZIUS PRESS

COMMON MISALIGNMENTS

- Feet, knees or hips asymmetrical
- Weight too far forward or back on feet, causing knee strain
- Abdomen sagging or lower back overarched
- Arms too far behind head, shoulders hunched, neck tense

ASSISTS

Beginners: As in Mountain Pose, stabilize the base first, working from bottom to top. Check for equal weight on feet, with equal weight distribution across all 4 corners of feet. Check to see the feet or ankles aren't rolling in toward each other. If so, bring attention to inner ankles and suggest a lifting up, or separate the heels ever so slightly. Feet, ankles, knees and hips are symmetrical and parallel. If legs appear too soft, have student separate feet and squeeze a block sideways between thighs. Tailbone still drops downward.

Beginners/Intermediate: From the side, look for and adjust extra arching or collapsing in lower back, which can put additional pressure on the knees. Tailbone lengthens down as inner thighs squeeze *together*—this helps to strengthen the center of gravity. *Mula* and *uddiyana bandhas* are great reinforcements here. Front ribs soften in.

Intermediate/Advanced: Standing behind, use the Seat Squeeze* to stabilize hips and pelvis. You can also straddle student's hips, steadying the base, then help bring torso into good alignment. Keep hips anchored as you lift up and support back ribs, massage tense shoulders and lengthen neck. Alternatively, have student gently sit on your thighs—this gives their legs a rest while you work on upper body. Once again, tailbone lengthens down, no arching in lower back.

Intermediate/Advanced: With great alignment in lower body, move on to these refinements. For example, move arms forward so hands are in line with heart. Rotate upper arms/biceps so that palms turn to face inward. Massage and press trapezius muscles down to create a release in the top of shoulders. Look for clean angles from feet to knees, knees to hips and hips to fingertips, with an overall lift through entire body. The position, even if deep, shouldn't "bottom out."

The Seat Squeeze is a fantastic stabilizing assist where you use both hands to firmly squeeze in outer hips/buttocks toward each other, anchoring in and down. From an anchored base, the student can then expand up or out in the energetic direction of the pose.

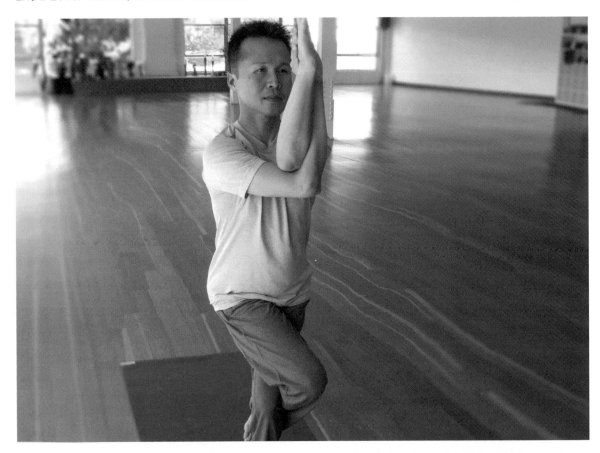

GARUDASANA—EAGLE POSE

The noblest of birds, it was an eagle—Garuda—who transported Lord Vishnu across the sky in the epic Indian story, The *Mahabharata*. If you've ever been lucky enough to see eagles in flight, their power and grace is unmistakable.

Eagle is a beautiful standing pose that should appear steady, balanced and light. The standing foot is stable, with even weight distribution. The outer hips/IT band must be adequately stretched for the legs to wrap around each other fully, with the lower knee ideally facing forward. Length in the side waist frees up the chest and shoulders. Even with modifications, beginners benefit greatly from this pose. It tones the legs, develops balance and delivers a terrific, bird-like sensation.

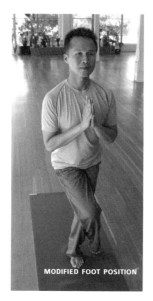

MODIFIED FOOT POSITION

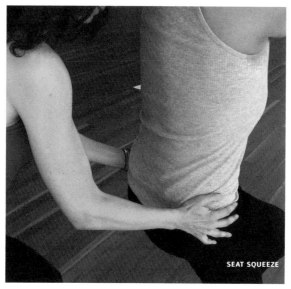

SEAT SQUEEZE

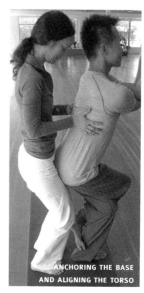

ANCHORING THE BASE
AND ALIGNING THE TORSO

COMMON MISALIGNMENTS

- Difficulty crossing knees, from tightness in legs or hips
- Base not strong—pelvic floor collapsed, inner thighs not squeezing in

- Torso too far forward, hips and shoulders out of linear alignment
- Shoulders hunched

ASSISTS

Beginners: As always, assist the base first to ensure a steady and balanced supporting leg. If student can't wrap foot behind calf, help them modify by placing foot on floor to the side of standing foot, or just cross thighs/knees in a stable position. Encourage the lower knee to square to front as much as possible. For tight shoulders, modify the arm position, elbows crossed at center of body, or hands in prayer position at the heart.

Beginners/Intermediate: From the side, look for and adjust over-arching or collapsing in lower back, which can put additional pressure on the supporting leg. Tailbone lengthens *down* while inner thighs squeeze together—reinforcing the center of gravity. With your hands, support and lift up at back ribs so that sides of waist lengthen. Gently rotate both shoulders open from the sides, if you see rounding in upper back, as elbows lift upward.

Intermediate/Advanced: Standing behind, use the Seat Squeeze to stabilize hips and pelvis. You can also straddle the student's hips and help to bring torso into good alignment relative to the hips (i.e. shoulders in line with hips, not rounded forward). Keep hips anchored as you lift up/support back ribs, massage tense shoulders and lengthen neck. Alternatively, have student gently sit on your thighs—giving their legs a rest—while you work on torso. *Drishti* (or gaze) for Eagle is over the fingertips, extending physical/spiritual vision outward.

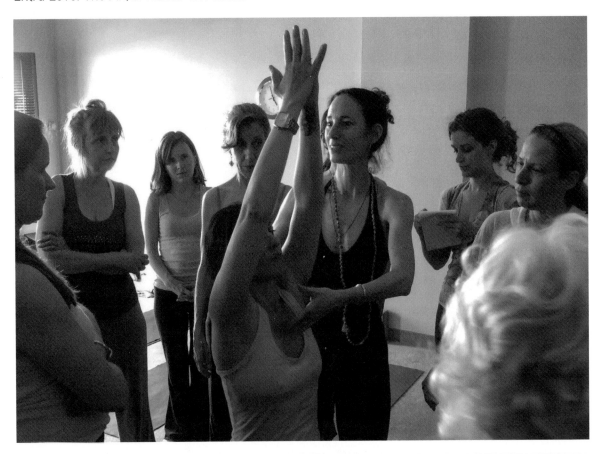

VIRABHADRASANA 1—WARRIOR 1 POSE

Virabhadra is one of the many deities associated with Lord Shiva. Facing disapproval from his father-in-law and loss of his beloved, Sati, Shiva plucked a hair from his head in a rage. He threw it to the ground and from that sprang Virabhadra, who redeemed Shiva's reputation and the reincarnation of his beloved.

In a fast-paced *vinyasa* class, the alignment of Warrior 1 is often confused with Warrior 2—the key difference being pelvis and chest squared forward to the front or side, respectively. You often see an in-between version, with the upper body trying to square to the front, while pelvis, torso and arms lean somewhat sideways. It's a tricky situation. When the pelvis swings opens to the side, the student loses alignment and strength in both legs.

Precise alignment and assists to Warrior 1, as simple as resetting the feet, make a big difference. Your assist should strive for even weight distribution on feet, correct foot pattern to allow for width and flexibility of hips and helping students achieve the general shape of the pose without collapsing the legs or lower back. Also aim to bring awareness to the back leg and entire back body.

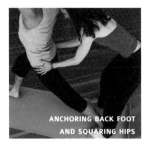
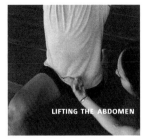
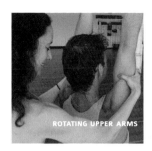
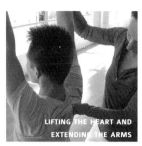

ANCHORING BACK FOOT AND SQUARING HIPS

LIFTING THE ABDOMEN

ROTATING UPPER ARMS

LIFTING THE HEART AND EXTENDING THE ARMS

COMMON MISALIGNMENTS

- Feet over-crossed, or edge of back foot peeling off floor, front knee rolling in/out
- Pelvis, torso and shoulders not squared to front

- Abdomen/lower back sagging—not enough effort to lift energy up
- Not going deep enough—hesitation due to weak legs or stiff hips
- Arms too far back

ASSISTS

Beginners: First, I always check the foot pattern. Classical alignment—front heel to back instep—requires good flexibility in the hips, back calf and Achilles tendon. Heel to instep alignment doesn't work for many students and in some cases, the feet may even be over-crossed. Reset feet a little wider—as wide as hip-width apart, from side to side. If right foot is forward, it's in front of right hip; back left foot is behind left hip. Each foot, in other words, has it's own "lane." From front to back, feet are about one leg-length apart, with even weight distribution. Correct any rolling in on back foot by bringing awareness to inner/outer edges of foot. You may need to reset the foot pattern again, move back heel further back, or shorten the whole stance until student feels even weight and strength through both legs. These assists help square the pose to the front, realigning the lower body.

Intermediate: Once foot pattern is aligned, stand behind student and gently anchor their back foot with your foot, then manually square hips to the front while keeping back foot secure. Moving around to the front, anchor the front foot and help to position front knee directly above front ankle. Ideal front leg position has thigh parallel to floor, shin perpendicular. As you do the assists, make sure student continues to lift up through lower back as tailbone moves down. If I see pinching in their lower back, I usually have student lean their torso forward slightly and then reset the arms overhead reaching for full extension, as chest lifts up. In the finished pose, they should feel their shoulders aligned directly over their hips.

From the side or front, create more of a lift *up* the front body to correct sagging in the lower abdomen or lower back. I often place a fingertip at *uddiyana bandha* and tell the student to lift *up*. Gently place your hands on the trapezius muscles as a reminder to relax the upper shoulders.

Intermediate/Advanced: Using both hands, lift up back ribs or place one hand behind the student's heart (between the shoulder blades) and encourage a lift *up*. Rotate upper arms firmly so palms spin to face inward (as in Urdhva Hastasana) and adjust arms alongside ears or move arms forward to relieve any shoulder tension. An imaginary, straight line connects a spot between shoulder blades, on the back, all the way to outstretched hands. Palms pressed together or left apart. If upper body alignment looks optimized but the legs still look weak or hesitant, I'll have student bend front knee more toward 90 degrees, while keeping back leg strong and front body lifted. Front knee stays right above ankle, shin perpendicular.

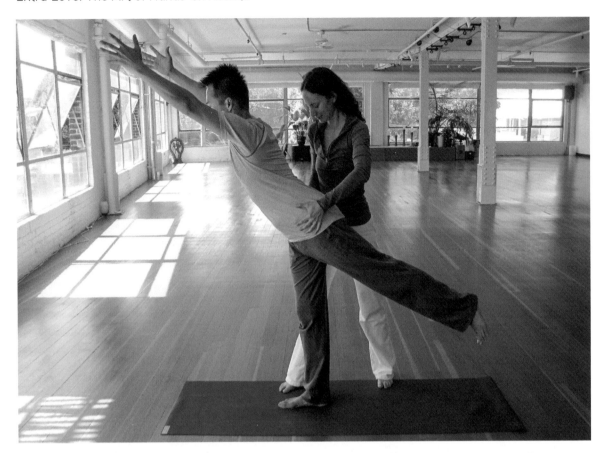

VIRABHADRASANA 3—WARRIOR 3 POSE

Warrior 3 requires steadiness, concentration and strength. Like Warrior 1, it brings tremendous awareness to the back body. The full pose has a long even shape: equal parts reaching forward and back, body parallel to floor. Beginners need help feeling balanced enough to tilt forward while lifting the back leg. Beginning and intermediate students benefit from stability at the middle of the pose—the center of gravity—from which they can expand out. Apply support first, then work on details. Even a light assist is very empowering.

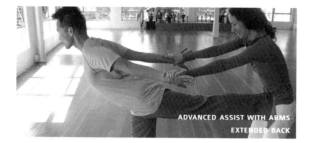

ADVANCED ASSIST WITH ARMS
EXTENDED BACK

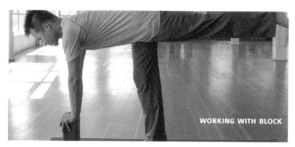

WORKING WITH BLOCK

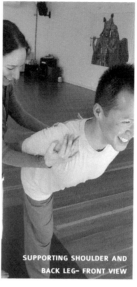

SUPPORTING SHOULDER AND
BACK LEG- FRONT VIEW

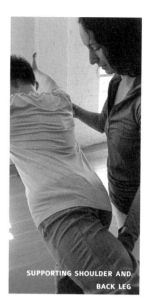

SUPPORTING SHOULDER AND
BACK LEG

COMMON MISALIGNMENTS

- Supporting leg unsteady
- Hips not level

- Lack of extension through legs, torso, arms

ASSISTS

Beginners: Help student find Tadasana in both legs as much as possible before transferring weight onto one leg. From arms-up position, have student practice tipping forward and back on one leg, feeling body come into a T shape. As they come forward into actual pose, stand to the side and give light support at the hips or front shoulder/back leg. For tight hamstrings, prop the hands up on a block, or use a small bend in front knee. In Warrior 3 with arms behind, which is easier on the lower back, steady the shape by supporting the front shoulder and back leg, encouraging square hips. These light assists help them find the essential shape of the pose.

Intermediate: Stand alongside supporting leg and provide steady support toward fuller back leg, torso and arm extension.

Advanced: A more advanced assist for Warrior 3—with arms extended behind—is for a solidly balanced student whose practice you know *well*. From behind, carefully take back foot and place it against your abdomen or hip, then take their wrists. Your approach must be steady and 100% confident! As their foot presses back into you, creating a resistance point, gently draw their arms longer behind, pulling back slightly. With the back leg anchored against you and arms securely held, they can expand out from the center to edges of pose.

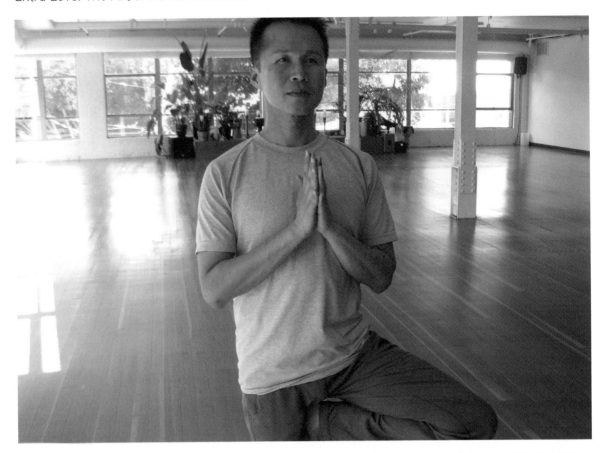

VRKSASANA—TREE POSE

Master Iyengar compares the eight limbs of Yoga to parts of a tree. *Yama*, the moral and ethical practices, are the roots. *Niyama*, the personal observances, correspond to the trunk. *Asanas*, performed with devotion, dedication and attention, are the branches. *Pranayama* corresponds to the leaves, breathing and aerating the whole form. *Pratyahara*, drawing the senses inward toward the soul, corresponds to the bark. *Dharana*, concentration, is represented by the sap or "juice" of the tree. *Dhyana*, meditation, corresponds to the flower. *Samadhi*, full integration of the whole being, is the fruit. Our spiritual development can be compared to the growth of a tree, from seed into maturity. The soul in each individual is what causes that individual to grow, just as the seed provides for growth of the tree. For a fruitful practice, all these parts come together.

Tadasana and Vrksasana have similar alignment characteristics. Comfort and confidence are important for the beginning student, whereas advanced students can be encouraged to lift up and "spread their branches." Assists in Tree Pose help students experience the pose's intrinsic, natural essence.

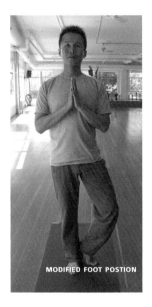
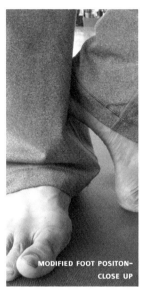
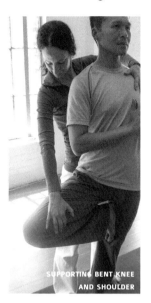
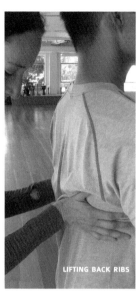

MODIFIED FOOT POSTION

MODIFIED FOOT POSITON– CLOSE UP

SUPPORTING BENT KNEE AND SHOULDER

LIFTING BACK RIBS

COMMON MISALIGNMENTS

- Balance off
- Working (bent knee) leg too turned out
- Lower back collapsed, not enough lift up front body

ASSISTS

Beginners: To help develop balance, start beginners with the working foot placed just inside supporting ankle, toes on floor, maintaining strength and lift through supporting leg. You can also have them practice standing on a block with one foot, holding steady. This really wakes up the standing leg. Use a wall for added support.

Beginners/Intermediate: In correct alignment, pelvis squares to the front in a neutral position. You may have to re-adjust the (working) bent knee leg, since often it's too turned-out to maintain alignment of pelvis. Working foot rests just *below* or *above* supporting knee, avoiding the knee joint. Notice foot placement and help student find a comfortable and safe position. When position looks secure, encourage a lifting up from the base, with chest also lifted. The pose should "grow" upward.

Intermediate: Check for lower back length: tailbone lengthens down as lower abdomen lifts up—similar to Tadasana assist—plus length through both side waists. Lift up and support back ribs. To support the entire shape, you can stand behind and close, supporting bent knee leg and opposite shoulder. Encourage extension and lift *up*.

Intermediate/Advanced: Use your toes to anchor student's supporting heel and your hands to lift up and support back ribs. The gentle occipital assist from Tadasana is also great here. Anchoring the heel roots them into the earth, as your hands help to grow the Tree taller. You should see a lovely lift up with these assists.

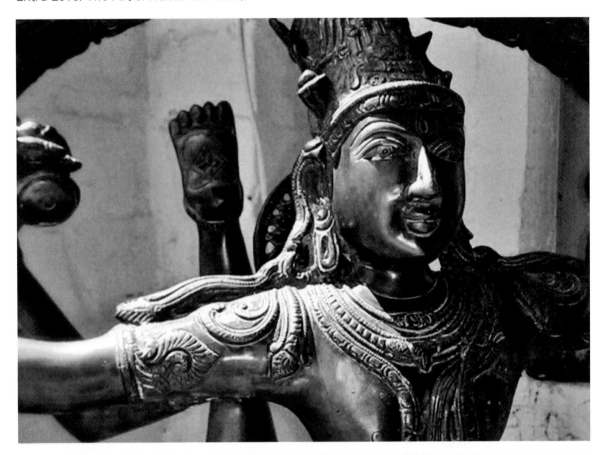

NATARAJASANA—DANCER POSE

From *nata* (dancer) and *raja* (lord), Nataraj is another name for Shiva, great master of dance. His dance is a metaphor for the continuous process of creation, preservation and destruction, the full cycle of life. Sculptures of Shiva Nataraj are recognizable in many yoga studios, his body surrounded by a circle of blazing fire.

Dancer Pose, a highlight of Bikram's Beginning Series, is equal parts standing pose, balance and back bend. As with Tree Pose, stability and balance are established in the standing leg. The arm lifts up to counterbalance the back leg. Hips stay level, the same distance from the ground. The back arches gracefully as the back leg extends up. Beginners need to develop good awareness in the supporting leg. Intermediate/advanced students benefit from light support so they can move deeper and fully extend the back leg. Once in the pose, the working hip often swings open to the side, which can destabilize alignment of the pelvis and throw balance off. The whole shape should appear steady and long, without twisting in the torso. Pelvis is neutral, ideally with no over-compression in the lower back.

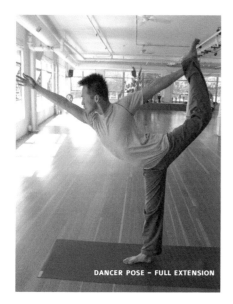
DANCER POSE – FULL EXTENSION

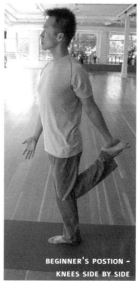
BEGINNER'S POSTION – KNEES SIDE BY SIDE

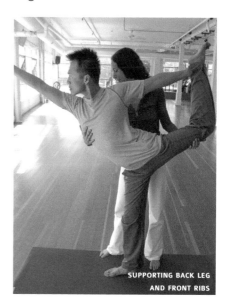
SUPPORTING BACK LEG AND FRONT RIBS

COMMON MISALIGNMENTS

- Foundation unsteady
- Working hip swings open, causing torso to twist
- Shoulders hunched

ASSISTS

Beginners: As in Tree Pose, help bring awareness and strength to supporting leg. Have student practice standing on a block with one foot. Returning to the floor, have them try coming into pose half-way, bending one knee to take the back foot, both knees aligned side by side, then switch sides, then hold one foot behind with both hands, switching sides. The idea is to stay balanced on the leg, with pelvis neutral and facing forward, torso vertical, no arch in lower back. Use the wall for extra support and/or a strap to extend reach.

Intermediate: Reinforce knee-to-knee alignment, then as foot draws away from pelvis, reinforce pressing into floor with standing foot, square pelvis and upward lift through whole body. Stand to side of supporting leg and steady the movement and provide support. If you notice sagging in lower abdomen, encourage a lifting *up* with a verbal cue or a light touch just below the navel (*uddiyana bandha*).

Intermediate/Advanced: Stand close on supporting leg side. Put one palm underneath front ribs, other palm underneath back thigh just above knee. As they progress up into position, this assist should simultaneously support and lift ribcage as back leg extends. Keep the torso lifted, sternum forward and up, back shin moving up and perpendicular to floor. To steady the base, gently anchor top of student's supporting foot with ball of your foot.

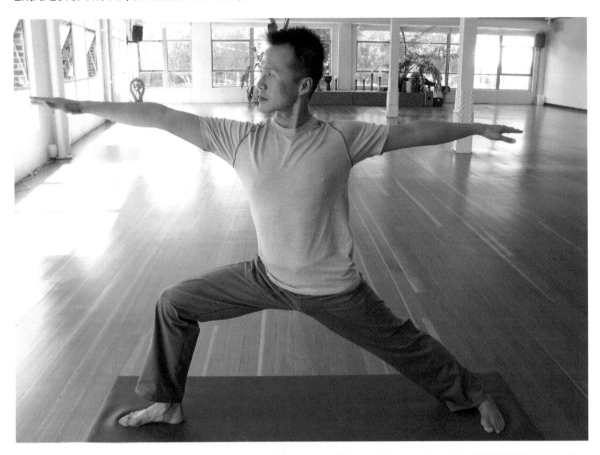

VIRABHADRASANA 2—WARRIOR 2 POSE

Moving from squared-hip to open-hip poses, we now get to Warrior 2. This is a gorgeous pose that helps students experience the interplay of opposites along with total body awareness. Whereas Warrior 1 alignment is often tricky for students, Warrior 2 is usually solid—students understand the shape very well. Beginners need help with basic alignment. Intermediate to advanced students enjoy additional refinement and strength.

Students' proficiency in Warrior 2 helps them execute many other poses: Reverse Warrior, Extended Side Angle, Balancing Half Moon and Triangle. You'll use similar assists for this entire family of standing poses.

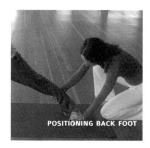
POSITIONING BACK FOOT

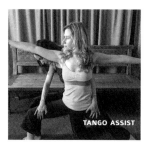
TANGO ASSIST

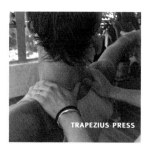
TRAPEZIUS PRESS

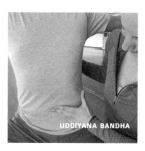
UDDIYANA BANDHA

COMMON MISALIGNMENTS

- Back foot turned out
- Front knee angles in or out
- Shoulders/torso leaning forward or back

- Collapse in abdomen or lower back—not enough effort to lift up
- Whole pose too rigid, needs to "breathe," shoulders tight

ASSISTS

Beginners: I talked about foot pattern in Warrior 1 and some of the same guidelines apply. From front to back, feet are about one leg-length apart or wider, with even weight distribution. Classical alignment of front heel to back instep is easier in Warrior 2. Nonetheless, look for and adjust if the feet over-cross (back foot stepped way behind pelvis, rather than aligned with front foot). Back foot turned in, heel reaching back, with back outer thigh lifting and hugging back, to keep outer edge of back foot anchored. Adjust collapsing of back thigh or rolling-in of back foot. You may have to shorten, or widen, the whole stance so student feels even weight/strength through both legs. Front knee, bent toward 90-degree angle, tracks directly over center of front foot, front thigh moving parallel to floor, shin perpendicular. Tailbone moves down.

Beginners/Intermediate: Work on refinements to upper body. Encourage a lift through torso, chest and back ribs, with equal length through sides of body. Arms parallel to floor, reaching equally away from center. Student should feel their shoulders directly over hips, as if the torso is shaped like a box. To experience more upper body expansion, you can belt the chest just below armpits and have student "breathe into" belt while holding the pose. This gives a great, full feeling throughout torso.

Intermediate: Once foot pattern is established, aim for lift and expansion. Check for sagging in lower abdomen and correct with light touch to *uddiyana bandha,* which helps lift abdomen and lighten legs. Sweep your hands up sides of body, for length and along arms, for expansion.

Intermediate/Advanced: Kneeling behind, your side body resting against student in a tango position, reach around and brace their back hip and front inner thigh. Use your body as a resistance point and pull their pelvis against you, to help externally rotate both legs. Check to see that front knee maintains a right angle with the lower ankle.

Manually, press trapezius muscles down and see that shoulder blades move down back. Help extend/lengthen arms from the biceps outward. Correct shoulders leaning forward or backward and reposition them directly over the hips. Lengthen neck and set head in a profile position, chin parallel to floor.

Advanced: Very flexible students tend to "sit" into back leg in Warrior 2 and Extended Side Angle. You'll see the back thigh/upper leg bowing toward floor. I always bring attention to this, lifting the back thigh a bit and sometimes resetting the back foot closer in. Back leg is strong and flexible, but not collapsed. A very strong back leg, incidentally, correlates to strength through *uddiyana bandha.*

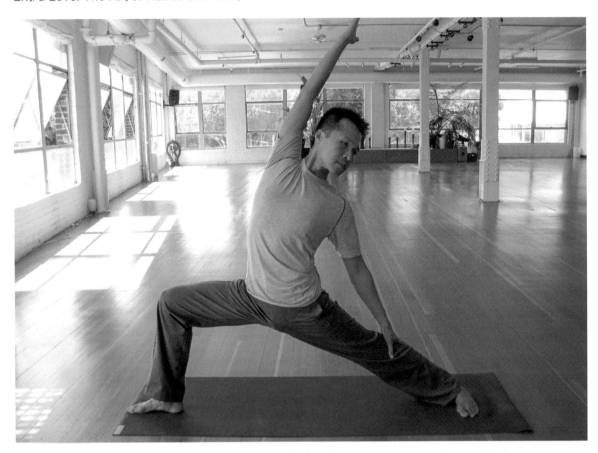

REVERSE WARRIOR POSE

One of my favorite standing poses, in this "reverse" version of Warrior 2 the foundation stays firm and solid. The torso remains spacious, facing to the side. The most common problem is collapsing or pinching in the lower back, right at the center of gravity. Warrior 2 is beautiful, but as soon as student reverses, the lower back tends to collapse. Your assist should aim for a deep side stretch, while fully and harmoniously integrating action of the upper and lower body.

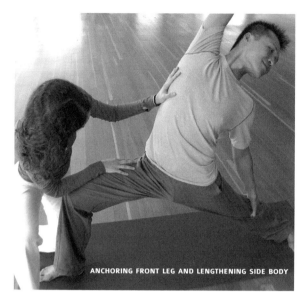

ANCHORING FRONT LEG AND LENGTHENING SIDE BODY

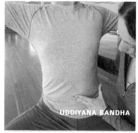

UDDIYANA BANDHA

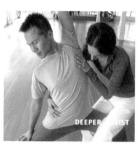

DEEPER ASSIST

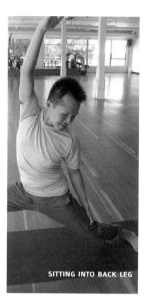

SITTING INTO BACK LEG

COMMON MISALIGNMENTS

- Too much weight in back leg, back foot collapsed
- Front knee rolls in

- Not enough lift in front body, collapsing lower back

ASSISTS

Beginners: As with Warrior 2, check the foot pattern and follow the same alignment guidelines. Bent front knee tracks directly over center of front foot. Adjust any rolling-in of front knee. Some beginners start with feet too close together, so I reset feet slightly wider apart to allow more "give" through the torso.

Beginners/Intermediate: Even with a good foot pattern, it's common to see sagging in lower abdomen. Very simply, you can assist with light touch to *uddiyana bandha* and tell the student to "lift HERE."

Intermediate: Once student is lifting up through center of gravity, stand or kneel just behind front leg, place one hand on front thigh, close to hip crease and provide firm anchoring/ resistance there. With your free hand or forearm, encourage lift and length through side body. The upper, reversing arm spirals inward, shoulder down. Your touch is firm but not forced; you'll sense either a gentle give or a slight resistance into the side bend. Go with what their body tells you.

Intermediate/Advanced: This is a deeper assist for strong students. Straddle the front leg firmly with your legs. Hook one hand behind lower side waist (closest to back leg), bracing other hand (or forearm) on upper side torso (closest to front leg). As you do the assist, three things happen: you actively *anchor* the front leg, lift *up* at the lower back/side waist and lift/ lengthen front side torso toward reversing position. For students with steady lower body alignment, this assist feels just fantastic. Adjust top arm with a gentle inner spiral, shoulder relaxed away from ear.

Advanced: Very flexible students tend to "sit" into back leg in Warrior 2, Extended Side Angle and Reverse Warrior. You'll see the back thigh/upper leg bowing toward floor. I always bring attention to this, lifting the back thigh a bit and sometimes resetting the back foot closer in. Back leg is strong and flexible, but not collapsed. A strong back leg, incidentally, correlates to strength through *uddiyana bandha*. Depth of pose is matched by core strength.

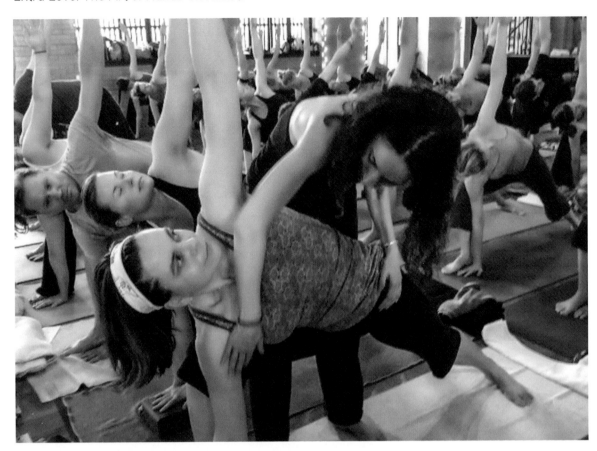

UTTHITA PARSVAKONASANA—EXTENDED SIDE ANGLE POSE

Extended Side Angle is a fantastic side body stretch, lower body aligning much like Warrior 2, upper body extending over front, bent knee. Ideal alignment is one straight line from back heel to top shoulder or fingertips of top hand. Two common issues to watch for are collapsing of torso forward, or collapsing of back leg. Many things are happening at once in this pose. Go for a strong, open shape with good alignment, body flat as in Triangle Pose, before taking students deeper.

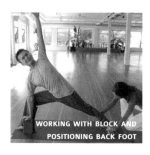
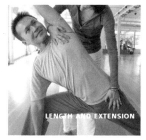
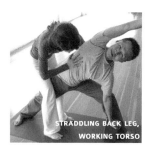
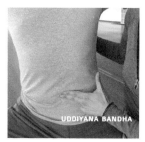

COMMON MISALIGNMENTS

- Front knee or back thigh collapse
- Torso collapses forward

- Shoulders hunched

ASSISTS

Beginners: Check foot pattern as you would for Warrior 2, front heel aligned to back instep, feet about one leg-length apart, weight evenly distributed. Back foot turned in, heel reaching back. Adjust rolling in on back foot. Bent, front knee tracks directly over center of front foot, front shin moves perpendicular to floor. For beginners, I often widen the stance, to create more space and "give" between the feet, facilitating the side stretch.

Have beginners place forearm on middle front thigh, or hand on a block, to keep an open shape through torso. Try to keep upper body weight from resting in lower shoulder; instead check that both shoulder blades move down the back. Upper arm extends straight up, or alongside ear with an inner spiral.

Intermediate: Aim for length and expansion. Stand behind, with your leg resting against back of student's front hip to anchor pelvis. From here, reach around and brace top hip open with one hand. With your free hand/forearm, help lengthen and rotate torso, or support opening across upper chest. As torso rotates, continue to use your leg as a resistance point from behind, keeping student's pelvis/back hip anchored. Make sure front knee maintains a right angle with lower ankle. From there, soften in front ribs and lengthen/support neck. Adjust any sagging in abdomen with light touch to *uddiyana bandha.*

Intermediate/Advanced: Deeper than assist above, straddle back leg close to hip, to anchor pelvis and manually rotate torso open and sideways, checking for good alignment through shoulders. You might even reach all the way under torso to initiate more rotation. This assist is effective for students in a very deep position, including a bind or half bind.

Advanced: Very flexible students tend to "sit" into back leg in Warrior 2, Reverse Warrior and Extended Side Angle. You'll see the back thigh/upper leg bowing toward floor. I always bring attention to this, lifting the back thigh a bit and sometimes resetting the back foot closer in. Back leg is strong and flexible, but not collapsed. A very strong back leg, incidentally, correlates to strength through *uddiyana bandha.*

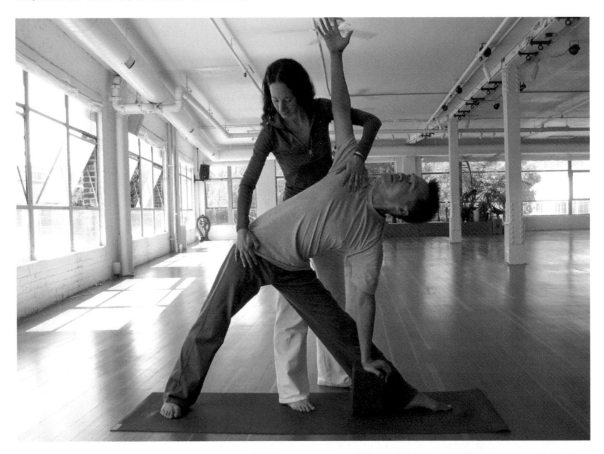

UTTHITA TRIKONASANA—TRIANGLE POSE

Renowned teacher Judith Lasater compares Triangle Pose to the archetype of a pyramid. Thousands of years old, it withstands the test of time because of its deep stability, connecting to earth while pointing to heaven. Master Iyengar describes Triangle as a great all-around pose for healthy functioning of the legs, hips and pelvis, stretching the back and chest, arms extending wide open. In the Sivananda tradition, Triangle is about space, feeling full extension through the whole body. Deep side body extension is emphasized in Bikram's version. My teacher Michael Carroll of Kripalu Yoga once said there is no "perfect" Triangle—each will reflect a student's body and particular energy. Your aim is to optimize and enhance what you see, with assists that are very similar to Warrior 2.

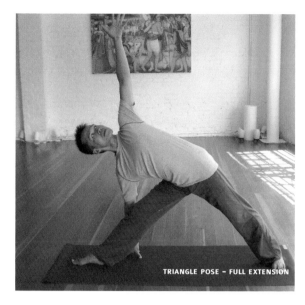

TRIANGLE POSE - FULL EXTENSION

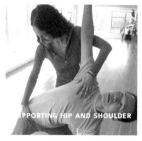

SUPPORTING HIP AND SHOULDER

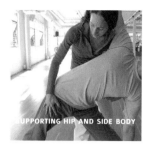

SUPPORTING HIP AND SIDE BODY

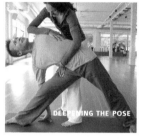

DEEPENING THE POSE

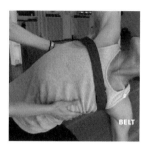

BELT

COMMON MISALIGNMENTS

- Foot pattern off—feet too close or over-crossed, uneven weight distribution
- Legs not activated

- Torso leaning forward
- Sitting into bottom shoulder, general collapsing of upper body

ASSISTS

Beginners: Check foot pattern—following assists for Warrior 2. Make sure the legs are activated, as in Mountain Pose, with kneecaps lifting, knees not hyper-extended. Front knee aligns on top of leg and does not roll in. Bring awareness to front thigh with a finger tap or light touch, so it stays strong and active. Both legs energetically spiral outward. As in Extended Side Angle Pose, I often widen the stance to make more space for torso's side bend.

Beginners/Intermediate: When you see the torso dropping forward, it usually means bottom hand is too far down. Reposition hand on a block or front shin—the raised position helps extend and activate the legs, bringing equal length to sides of body. Torso and back body come into alignment, as if pressed back against a wall. The seat should not stick out. Look for collapsing in bottom shoulder—common in Side Angle Pose, too—and help student roll shoulder open, away from ear. For a tight upper shoulder, reposition hand on hip. Belting the upper chest also feels great and helps student feel expansion through upper torso.

Intermediate/Advanced: Go for more expansion. From the back, standing hip to hip with student, put one hand around top hip, opposite hand reaching around to shoulder/upper chest area. The action of your hands is to anchor the pelvis, maintain its external rotation while lengthening side body from top hip to upper side of chest. Alternatively, put one hand on top hip, other hand *underneath* body at the upper back ribs, just below shoulder, to help expand and lengthen lower side waist. In half-bound or bound Triangle, you might reach all the way around torso to encourage deeper opening in the pose, upper shoulder braced for support.

Finishing touches: Lengthen arms, expand shoulder to shoulder/hand to hand and encourage length from tailbone to crown of head. Support and lengthen the neck. Direct gaze upward toward top hand.

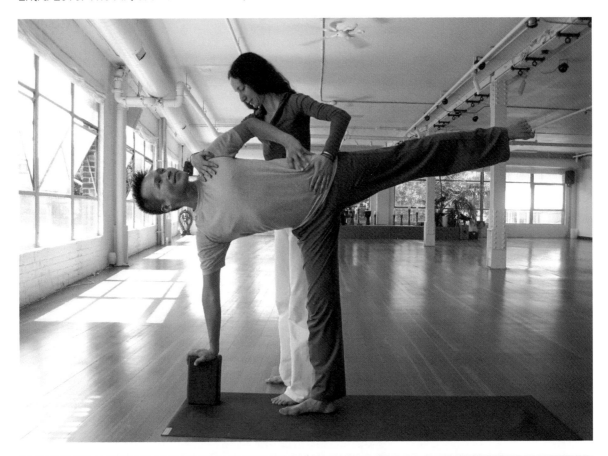

ARDHA CHANDRASANA—BALANCING HALF MOON POSE

Chandra means "shining moon," and refers to the lunar deity Soma, whose story is told in the *Vedas*. Young, beautiful and fair, Soma rides his chariot—the moon—across the night sky, pulled by ten white horses. All phases of the moon are said to be beneficial, the bright moon carrying the highest blessing.

The last of our open-hipped standing poses, Ardha Chandrasana—half standing pose, half balance—is structurally similar to Triangle Pose, just as Rotated Half Moon relates to Rotated Triangle. The pose calls for a steady base through the supporting leg/hand, from which the student can shine outward. Effective assists steady the base while reaffirming a clear connection between the lower and upper body. The hips and shoulders are evenly stacked. Often a simple assist—raising the floor up with a block— makes all the difference in the world. Your assists will be almost identical to Warrior 2 and Triangle, since the same principles apply. Apply support first, bring awareness to back body, then work on details.

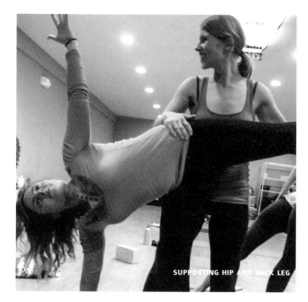
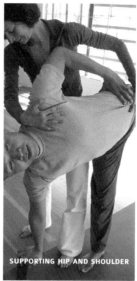
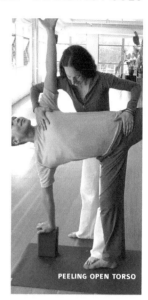

SUPPORTING HIP AND BACK LEG   SUPPORTING HIP AND SHOULDER   PEELING OPEN TORSO

COMMON MISALIGNMENTS

- Leg muscles not fully activated, especially supporting leg
- Energy stuck in lower body, not lifting up

- Upper hip rolls forward, usually relates to lower hand placed too far down
- Back body not expanded

ASSISTS

Beginners: As with Triangle, set a proper foundation using a block to raise floor up and reposition bottom hand so it's securely grounded. The modified hand position helps student extend and activate supporting leg. Student's opposite hand can go on top hip, as they start to come into pose. Steady them from behind, gently supporting/stabilizing hips, front shoulder/ upper chest and back leg. Encourage student to breathe deep and relax, as the pose can be overwhelming to newcomers.

Intermediate/Advanced: Standing close behind, gently anchor standing foot with ball of your own foot, stabilize and stack hips one on top of the other and "peel" open the torso from top shoulder to top hip, fully extending spine parallel to floor. Arrange and lengthen top arm directly over shoulder and encourage student to reach up.

Advanced: Work on the details—fully extended back leg, parallel to floor, back foot flexed. Side waist, torso and chest lengthening away from pelvis, equal length in both sides of body. Legs, torso and arms reach dynamically from the center. Neck in line with spine.

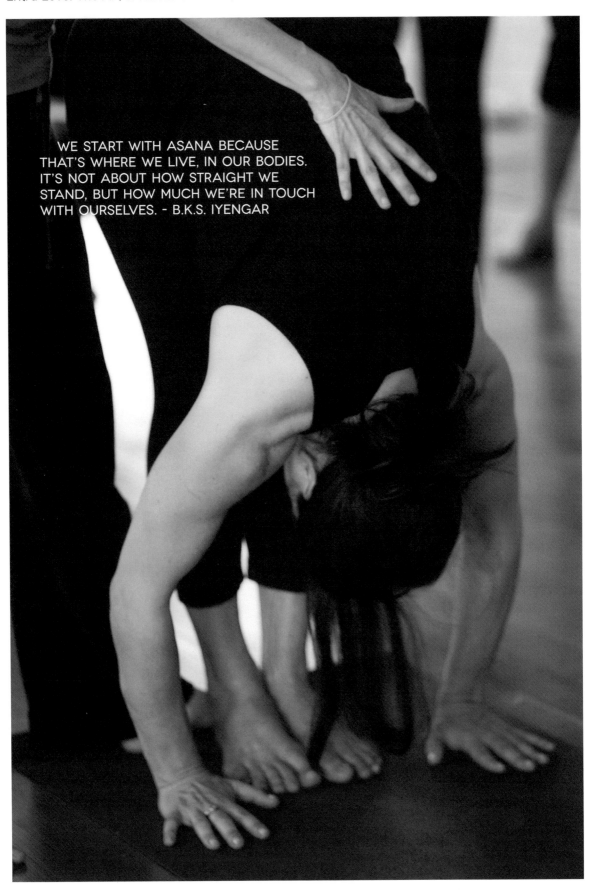

WE START WITH ASANA BECAUSE
THAT'S WHERE WE LIVE, IN OUR BODIES.
IT'S NOT ABOUT HOW STRAIGHT WE
STAND, BUT HOW MUCH WE'RE IN TOUCH
WITH OURSELVES. - B.K.S. IYENGAR

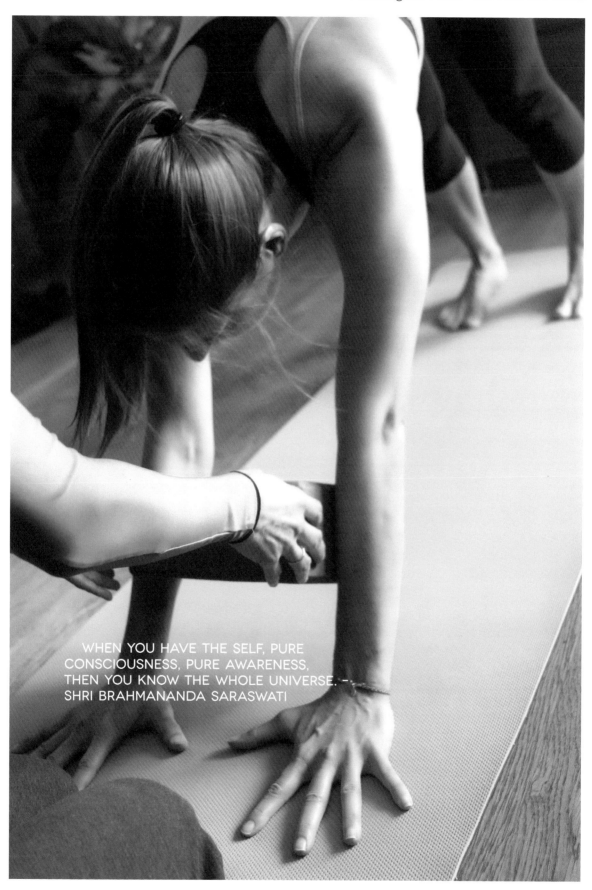

WHEN YOU HAVE THE SELF, PURE
CONSCIOUSNESS, PURE AWARENESS,
THEN YOU KNOW THE WHOLE UNIVERSE. -
SHRI BRAHMANANDA SARASWATI

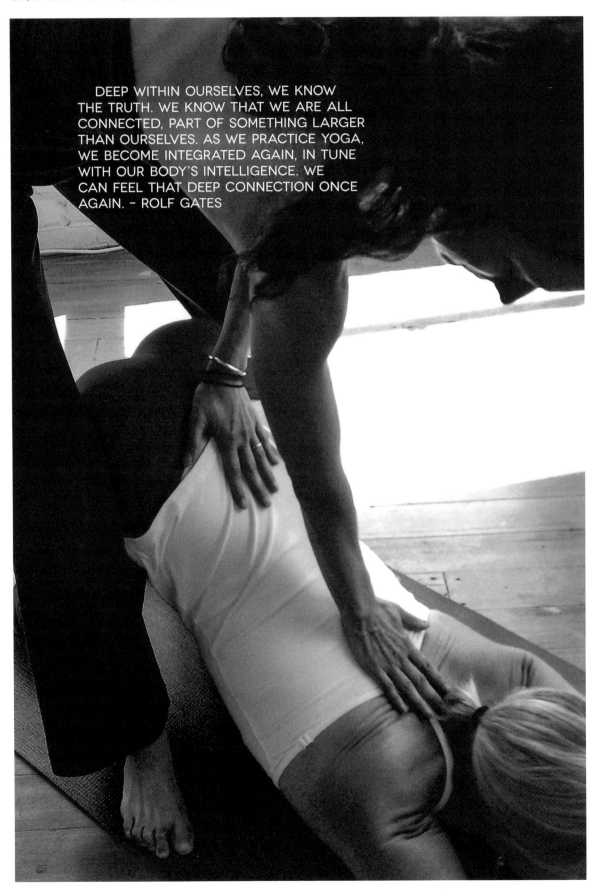

DEEP WITHIN OURSELVES, WE KNOW
THE TRUTH. WE KNOW THAT WE ARE ALL
CONNECTED, PART OF SOMETHING LARGER
THAN OURSELVES. AS WE PRACTICE YOGA,
WE BECOME INTEGRATED AGAIN, IN TUNE
WITH OUR BODY'S INTELLIGENCE. WE
CAN FEEL THAT DEEP CONNECTION ONCE
AGAIN. - ROLF GATES

BACK BENDS

Many teachers describe back bends as moving us into the future, since releasing the front body—the pelvis, psoas, chest and heart—is important if we are to move forward fearlessly and gracefully. In *EXTRA LOVE: Volume 1*, I talked about forward bends as our most habitual movements in daily life. Back bends, on the other hand, counterbalance our normal stance throughout the day. They are said to give energy and courage and to fight depression. One of my teachers in San Francisco says that if you are ever depressed or sad, back bends will make you feel better instantly.

The positioning of the feet and knees is important for all back bends. Students must learn how to anchor through the legs and pelvis with proper alignment, gradually inviting the spine, chest and shoulders to open from this foundation. This takes time and patience. Eventually, the energy and arch of the back bends move evenly through the spine. When assisting, it's especially important to stay sensitive to resistance points. Never fight on an assist. In many cases, relaxing muscles around the spine is the first step toward a deeper, then stronger, position.

In this section, I've organized the back bends into three groups, which generally speaking I'd classify as light, moderate and deep. The lighter back bends are Cobra Pose, variations on Locust Pose, Fish Pose and the arching action of Cat/Cow. Moderate back bends include Puppy Stretch, Bow Pose, Half Wheel Pose, Camel, Upward Facing Dog and "Wild Thing." The deeper back bends are Full Wheel and King Pigeon. These are general groupings only. Your students may have a different experience within the poses.

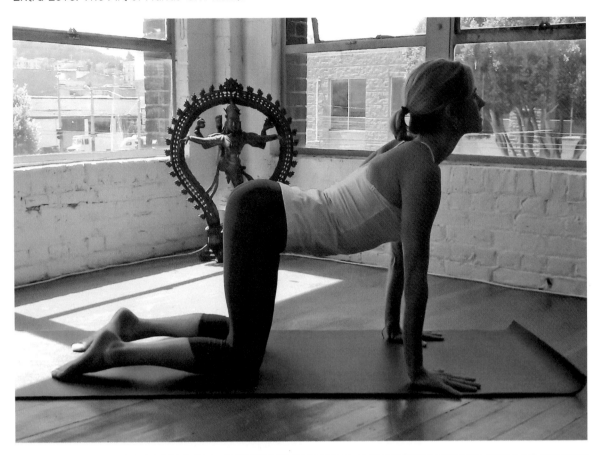

CAT/COW

Cat/Cow is one of my favorite warm-up stretches, a light back bend combining arching *and* rounding of the spine. For beginners, it's often their first entrée into back bending poses and the first time they will feel full articulation–contraction and extension—of the spine. As simple as the stretch is, misalignments are common in Cat/Cow, for example, unconscious placement of the hands, arms, legs or torso. Good assists and adjustments bring awareness and symmetry into the whole body, giving students a solid foundation for Cobra, Upward Facing Dog, Anantasana/Puppy Stretch, Downward Facing Dog, Sphinx Pose and arm balances such as Plank Pose.

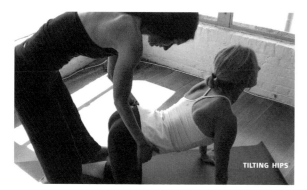

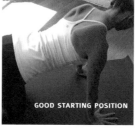

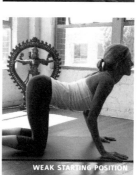

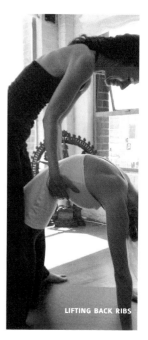

COMMON MISALIGNMENTS

- Hands/feet misplaced
- Collapsing of shoulders or lower back, which can carry into Downward Facing Dog
- Uneven curvature in back during arching/rounding action

ASSISTS

Beginners: Set up beginners in a good starting position. From Table Pose (hands/knees position), hands are shoulder distance apart, wrists just under shoulders, bent knees are hip-width apart just under hips. Typical weak spots in Table Pose—in arms, shoulders or middle to lower back—are important to point out to new students. Hands spread out and press into floor with no sagging in wrists, arms actively extend and stretch energetically away from floor. Shoulders wrap onto upper back as upper arms rotate externally from the "inside out." As student moves into Cat/Cow, look for a nice, even curve along the spine. You may notice places where the curvature doesn't seem even, for example, the lower back arches deeply but middle back is quite stiff. These are clues for assisting effectively.

Beginners/Intermediate: To help the arching/rounding action, stand behind and gently tilt the hips back as student arches, then lift firmly underneath the middle rib cage during the rounding position. Your assist aims to even out both actions, arching and rounding. Make sure neck stays in line with spine, to help protect the delicate bones of the cervical spine. Sagging in the neck sometimes indicates that hand/foot pattern is off, hands too far forward or knees too far back. Double-check the starting position.

Advanced: Refine the alignment further, going for an absolutely even curve in the back, with good range of motion in thoracic or middle spine. Arms are fully activated and extended, muscles hugging to the bone. Strong and active arms in this pose suggest the support needed for Plank Pose, Side Plank, Handstand and other arm balances.

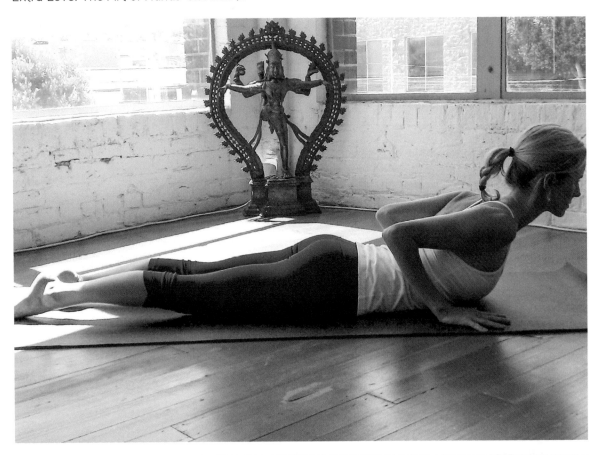

BHUJANGASANA – COBRA POSE

In *Jivamukti Yoga: Practices for Liberating Body and Soul*, my teachers Sharon and David include a beautiful passage on Bhujangasana. Important mythological icons in Yoga, cobras are said to be attracted to beings of high attainment. Shiva wears snakes around his neck and body and *kundalini*—individual consciousness—is represented as a snake. When *kundalini* is awakened, she is attracted upward toward her celestial lover, Shiva, residing at the third eye. *Kundalini's* ascent toward her lover is a metaphor for our own consciousness moving from ignorance to bliss. As a gateway to other back bends, the symbolism and importance of Cobra Pose are beautiful to behold.

Cobra is a light back bend, yet students often make it more difficult through confusion with Upward Facing Dog. They are closely related but not identical. Assists in Cobra should aim for a shape and experience that helps distinguish the two poses. I often remind students that Cobra, the snake, remains close to the ground, pelvis and navel staying on the floor. Effective assists bring awareness and consciousness to the entire back body. Students with alignment, poise and confidence in Cobra can more easily progress upward toward High Cobra (extending the arms more) and Upward Facing Dog.

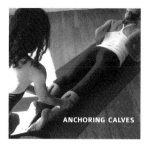
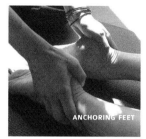
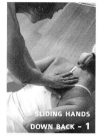
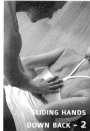
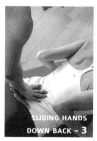
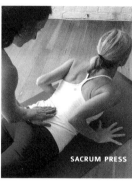
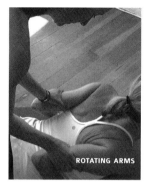
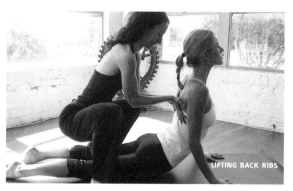

COMMON MISALIGNMENTS

- Confusion with Upward Facing Dog, causing compression in lower back
- Legs soft or too far apart
- Limited back or arm strength, causing collapsing in chest or upper body
- Hands too far forward, elbows too wide, or shoulders hunched

ASSISTS

Beginners: Set up good alignment, legs parallel and together, tops of feet on floor, toes spread, quadriceps active but buttocks relaxed, pelvis and navel resting on floor. Hands placed flat so wrists align under elbows, arms bent at roughly ninety degrees. Shoulder blades move down the back as elbows squeeze toward the midline. Encourage a slow, gradual approach to Cobra, leading up with the heart, rather than chin or shoulders. Neck is soft and gaze is straight ahead or slightly downward. Let beginners come up as high as possible without using their hands to gauge their back strength, then press up using hands.

Beginners/Intermediate: With good alignment in place, there are several good assists to create more sensation and strength. Anchor feet or lower calves as student lifts up into and holds pose, so they feel back body working. Also, with your hands side by side or overlapping, slide your palms from the back of heart to sacrum, drawing a clear line of energy down the back. Or stand behind and lightly lift/support back ribs as in Warrior 1. To create awareness and lift in the chest, use a press point at the sternum and cue student to lift up, pressing their hands firmly into floor. These assists bring good awareness to legs, pelvis, back body and upper chest.

Intermediate: Moving on to somewhat stronger assists, stand or squat above and stack your hands—palms facing down—on top of sacrum, then root down with your hands and draw back firmly. Your action lengthens tailbone back and frees up chest to lift higher. Also standing behind, grip biceps firmly and externally rotate the inner upper arms from the inside out, grounding the triceps back and down. This assist draws open the shoulders and upper chest and feels fantastic.

Advanced: More advanced students are able to lift chest higher into High Cobra. Here, you can give a passive assist by anchoring the feet/calves. Standing behind, you can also support and lift up the back ribs. Make sure upper body alignment stays steady. Arms hug in, elbows squeeze toward each other, shoulders down as shoulder blades move down the back. Look for even curvature in spine. To prevent compression or a "break" in lower back, encourage extra length back through tailbone.

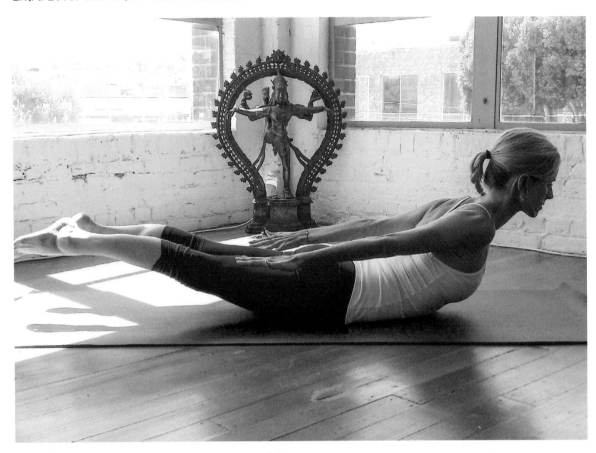

SALABHASANA – LOCUST POSE

Salabhasana is a light to moderate back bend that requires a bit more back body contraction and strength than Cobra Pose. A phenomenally beneficial pose, Locust is great for beginners. The stronger the back gets, the higher students can lift up.

There are several great variations of Locust among the different styles of Yoga. Misalignments are rare, usually reflecting simple weakness in the legs or back muscles. The legs remain as parallel as possible, helping to protect the lower back as the chest initiates the movement upward. Think of the legs as a tail, the shoulders as wings.

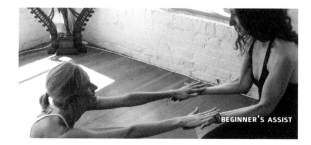
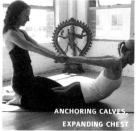
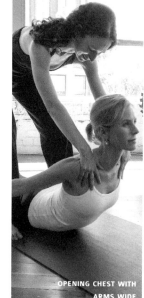
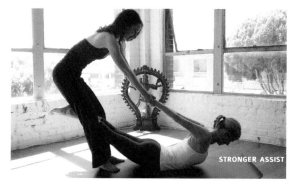
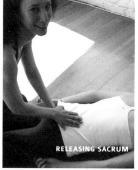

BEGINNER'S ASSIST

ANCHORING CALVES, EXPANDING CHEST

STRONGER ASSIST

RELEASING SACRUM

OPENING CHEST WITH ARMS WIDE

COMMON MISALIGNMENTS

- Upper chest dropped, not enough strength to lift up
- Lack of lifting action in legs
- Neck compressed

ASSISTS

Beginners: In arms-extended-forward variation, kneel in front and place your hands under student's palms. Provide steady support and lift until their feet just begin to drop. Then have them hold position on their own. If you see tension in the neck or shoulders, have student drop chin, draw shoulder blades down the back and gaze slightly downward. This is a gentle, fun assist for beginners.

Intermediate: In hands-clasped-behind variation, anchor feet/calves as in Cobra. For further lift, gently sit on student's calves, take their wrists and draw their arms back slightly to help expand front chest. You're assisting just enough to lift and open the chest, but *not so much* that the lower back compresses.

Intermediate: In arms-wide-airplane variation, stand behind and use your hands to gently lift and open the upper chest area, drawing back at about a forty-five degree angle. Again, you're assisting just enough to open the chest, but not so much that lower back pinches.

Intermediate/Advanced: Here's a stronger assist, where you use your legs and hands to help extend and lift up. From behind, step around student's calves with your heels close in, feet turned out, knees bent (in ballet, this is first position, *demi plié*). Take student's shins and wedge them between your calves. Take their wrists with your hands, making sure their palms face in. In one smooth, *even* action, draw their lower body long and back by leaning back and squeezing slightly with your legs, as you simultaneously pull back on wrists, drawing their upper chest open. Elongate the whole shape on a *diagonal line* reaching *back*, lifting up chest with no lower back compression. The assist gives a feeling of liftoff, as the Locust takes flight.

All levels: In the one-legged variation of Locust, make sure the neck is aligned with spine: chin, mouth or forehead resting on floor, arms underneath body. For the assist, slide one hand under working thigh to lift it up slightly, as your other hand rests firmly on the sacrum, rooting tailbone down.

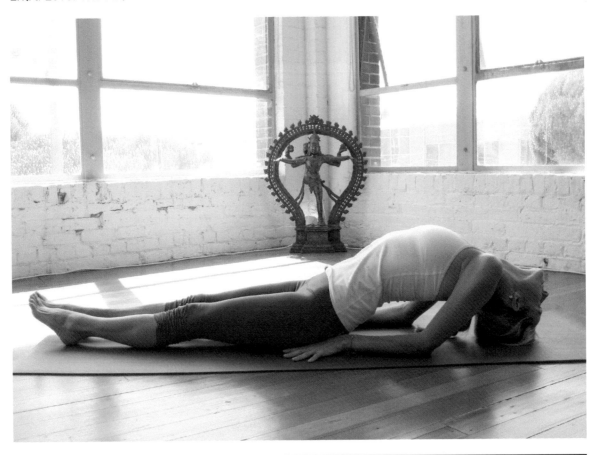

MATSYASANA – FISH POSE

Matsyasana is the asana dedicated to Matsya, the fish incarnation of Lord Vishnu, maintainer of the universe and all creatures. Once upon a time the whole earth was in danger of a disastrous flood. Vishnu took the form of a fish, saving humanity along with the sacred teachings known as the *Vedas*. Today, many of the ocean's wild fish are close to extinction from overfishing, giving the pose new meaning and potency. This is a beautiful pose, with the heart lifted higher than the rest of the body.

Fish is a light back bend, easy for most beginners, but challenging for students with rounding in the upper back, scoliosis, history of neck injury, or a heavily muscled torso. It tones the back body and serves as a counter pose to Shoulder Stand and Plow Pose. Minimal assists to the upper body help most students rise up into Fish with a full and open heart.

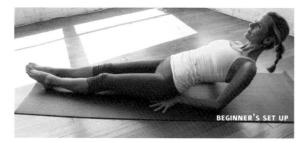
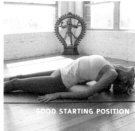
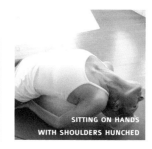
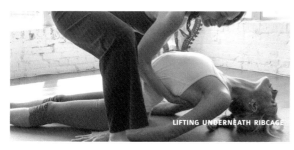
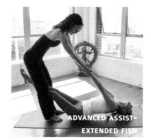
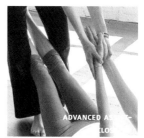

COMMON MISALIGNMENTS

- Hands too far back
- Shoulders shrugging up
- Chest collapsed
- Lower back compression

ASSISTS

Beginners: Familiarize students with basic shape and how to get into pose. Start seated with legs out, leaning back on forearms. The pelvis tilts forward as they puff up chest, shoulder blades scooping together behind back. Hands inch down toward thighs, as chest lifts and top of head comes toward floor. If student can't stay on forearms without collapsing chest, use a rolled up blanket or block under upper back, placed sideways about level with shoulder blades. Added support under the head helps protect the neck. Use sternum press or touch to encourage lift in upper chest.

Beginners/Intermediate: Students love to sit on their hands in Fish. In most cases, this throws off alignment of the torso, caves in the chest and shrugs shoulders up by the ears. I usually encourage hands alongside of body. It's easy to adjust—just have student take hands out from under seat, walk hands *forward* toward mid-thighs, keeping elbows bent by side body. They may need to shift a few times before finding a good position, with secure arms and heart lifting up. Repositioning of the hands almost *always* improves alignment of upper body. If the chest still collapses, call in a prop (e.g., rolled blanket) for extra support.

Intermediate: Once student is comfortable in pose, you want the back muscles relaxed, spine pulling up toward center of the body. Standing above, reach your hands underneath ribcage. With your palms facing up, lift up and cradle student's upper back for a couple of breaths. Their head comes only slightly off floor—if at all—and definitely no more than about a half inch. Let the back bend "blossom" there as you give support, then gently release head back down to original position. After the assist, you'll see that the chest has more lift. For a deeper assist, just as you lift upper back, massage along either side of spine, holding torso up with your elbows. Be careful not to place any pressure directly on the spine; work just to either side. Then place the head back down gently.

Advanced: For extended Fish, this assist is similar to the Intermediate/Advanced assist for Locust Pose, only instead of facing down, the student is facing up. Stand in front and secure student's shins with your legs as you take hold of wrists. Draw student toward you, pulling back gently with your legs and hands, lengthening the whole shape on a diagonal line reaching *back*. The chest is lifting, with no lower back compression.

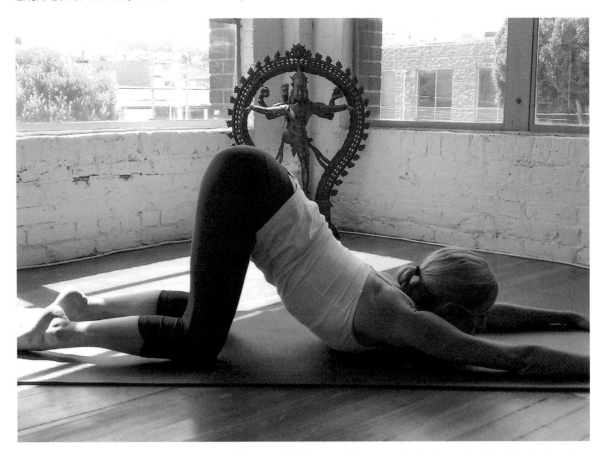

ANANTASANA—PUPPY STRETCH AND KNEES/CHEST/CHIN

Anantasana, also called Puppy Stretch, is named for Ananta, or *Shesh Nag,* the serpentine seat of Lord Vishnu. As a light-to-moderate back bend accessible to all levels, Puppy Stretch is great as a transition in between standing poses or deeper back bends,or as a restorative pose. Held for several breaths, the pose is deeply therapeutic.

Good practice with Cat/Cow prepares students for the pose. Assists help beginning students find the general shape, developing flexibility in the spine as preparation for deeper back bends. Advanced students tend to overarch the back, which you can adjust with a few simple assists.

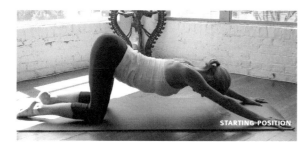
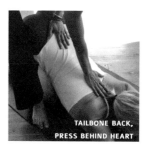
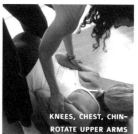
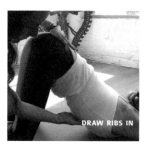
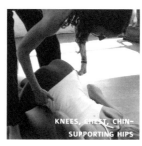
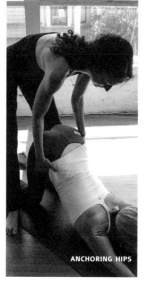

COMMON MISALIGNMENTS

- Hips not aligned over bent knees, or knees too wide
- Lower back or shoulders compressed

ASSISTS

Beginners: Build a good foundation, starting on hands and knees and gradually walking hands forward. Knees, shins and feet hip-width apart, parallel, with hips right above bent knees. Symmetry of knees and shins helps prevent compression in lower back and sacrum. Students with tighter shoulders can rest up on the hands or elbows. Watch for shoulders hunching. Hug them back away from ears if needed.

Intermediate: Once forehead or chest is on floor, stand around hips to anchor them in place, as you gently press a hand in between shoulder blades behind the heart. Emphasize length between hips and heart. As with beginners, watch for shoulder compression or pinching in lower back. Keep tailbone moving straight back, with a gentle pull back on sacrum. Check to see ribs are softening into front body when you step away from assists.

Advanced: Very flexible students tend to overarch the lower back here and in Downward Facing Dog. While it may feel great, overarching can lead to structural instability in the lower back and/ or chronic lower back pain. I use the assist above—tailbone moving *back*, front ribs drawing in, *uddiyana bandha activated*—and encourage a long, strong shape.

A variation on Puppy Stretch, Knees/Chest/Chin has similar assists. Stand above and lift and support hips as student lowers down; once chest is down, apply same assist as Cobra. Hold biceps firmly and externally rotate upper arms, moving elbows toward each other behind the back. This helps to draw open shoulders and upper chest. With hips anchored with your legs, as in Puppy Stretch, place one hand between shoulder blades, behind the heart, to encourage a release/softening in upper back.

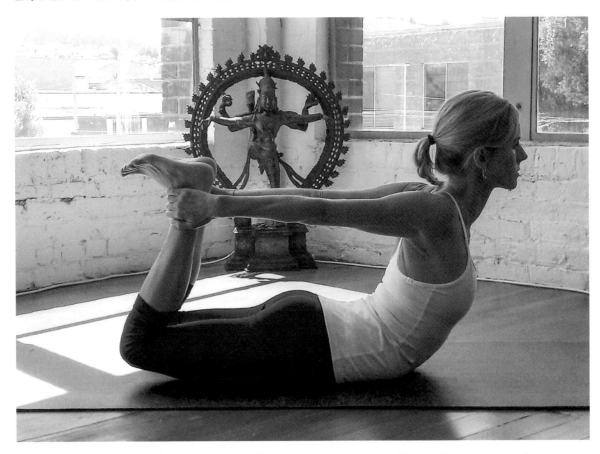

DHANURASANA – BOW POSE

Dhanurasana is in many ways the most challenging moderate back bend leading up to Full Wheel. In the pose, we experience an untapped reserve of potential energy as we stretch open the front of the body as the feet draw up high behind. The sensation is like pulling an arrow back in a bow, arms taut like strings, the rest of body making a bow shape. After the release, Bow Pose sends a rush of energy into the entire body.

Students may have difficulty with the pose at first. The legs might start out wide, the chest close to the floor. Once they come up, if too much of the arch concentrates in the lower back, students can lose evenness and power. There should be a nice, even arch through the spine, with equal parts pulling (with the hands) and kicking back (with the feet), so the bow shape draws evenly through the torso. Be prepared with props, creative problem-solving and plenty of encouragement for beginners.

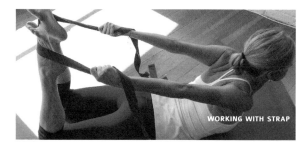
WORKING WITH STRAP

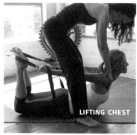
LIFTING CHEST

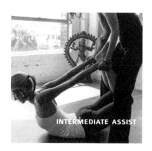
INTERMEDIATE ASSIST

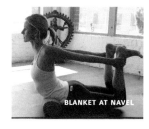
BLANKET AT NAVEL

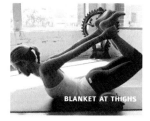
BLANKET AT THIGHS

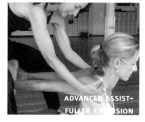
ADVANCED ASSIST-
FULLER EXTENSION

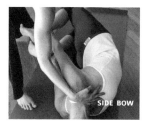
SIDE BOW

COMMON MISALIGNMENTS

- Quadriceps or shoulders tight—difficulty reaching feet
- Lower back compressed, with knees far apart

- Uneven shape: not enough pulling action from hands or kicking back with feet
- Neck or shoulders hunched

ASSISTS

Beginners: Set up initial position with knees hip-width apart or wider. Help student reach feet with a strap, if needed. Allow them to come into pose gradually, lengthening thighs as knees bend. Chest (rather than chin, neck or shoulders) leads the pose, moving forward and up. Encourage a nice, even curve through entire body, weight centered on pelvis and abdomen, equal efforts kicking back with legs and pulling with hands. If chest collapses toward floor—but you sense they could lift up higher—give a light, pressing assist on the sternum. Encourage them to lift UP as they pull back even more with the hands. Gently reach around shoulders/upper chest and provide very *light* support. Check for active legs, front body lifting, knees and shoulders about equal distance from floor.

Intermediate: For students with good, symmetrical alignment, give a stronger assist aimed at extending and opening front of body, deepening the back bend. Stand just above and place your feet around the lower, outer thighs to keep their legs parallel and anchored. Reach down and firmly grasp around the student's wrists, close to where heels meet hands. From here, gently and evenly draw straight UP. As soon as you start to lift, you'll immediately sense a resistance point, where the back won't naturally arch without compression. *Don't go any higher.* Stay steady, allowing student to breath deep and absorb the assist.

Intermediate/Advanced: Here are a few assists to help students experience arching throughout the spine. You need a blanket and a block. First, roll up blanket and put it sideways, just at the navel. Lifting into Bow Pose, the rolled blanket transfers weight *back* onto thighs, for a fuller opening in upper body. The rolled blanket, placed sideways at thigh crease, transfers weight *forward* for more extension through the legs. These variations help students experiment with weight shifting forward and back. A block, placed sideways just under lower ribs, helps to boost up the torso, so legs are temped to kick even higher. It feels great, so long as there's no lower back compression. The block is my favorite prop for Bow Pose.

Advanced: This assist goes for fuller extension in upper body. Carefully take a squatting position and "sit" gently on top of the student's flexed feet, anchoring the legs. As you make contact, reach around to where shoulders meet upper chest. Lean back slightly, anchoring legs back and down and help to raise chest higher. Their thighs remain *on the floor.* This assist is ideal for students with a deeper arch in their back, strong *uddiyana bandha*, feet clearly flexed up and no habit of lower back compression.

For Parsva Dhanurasana (Side Bow), gently support around top shoulder/upper chest and back thigh, just above the knee, as they breathe deeply into pose. Head angles toward floor, neck relaxed. Students in this version should have good symmetry in the legs, even arch in the spine and secure grip on feet or ankles.

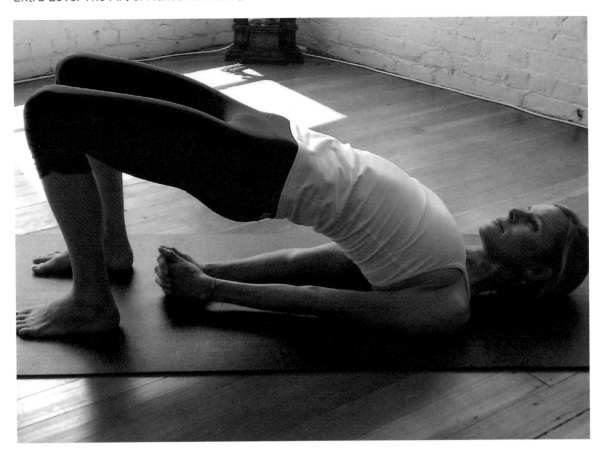

SETU BANDHASANA – BRIDGE POSE OR HALF WHEEL

Moving closer to Urdhva Dhanurasana, Full Wheel Pose, we have Bridge Pose, or Half Wheel. Structurally, Bridge is very similar to Camel Pose and the same alignment guidelines apply. Students learn how to anchor through the legs and pelvis with proper alignment, gradually inviting the spine, chest and shoulders to open from this foundation.

As a moderate back bend, Bridge Pose is accessible to beginning through advanced students. The most common challenge here is lack of strength or awareness in the feet and legs, which propel the back bend action from the floor up through the spine, rather than flexibility in the spine itself. The shoulders might also be tight, preventing the arch from moving up the torso. Several great assisting and prop options work for different levels and body types so that all students can have a great experience in this pose. Like other back bends, go for a nice, even curve throughout the spine. As my teachers have said, Bridge Pose is a metaphor for how we might connect our lower level of consciousness to our higher, divine Self.

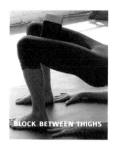
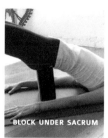
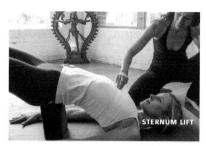
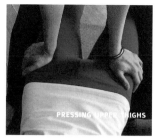

BLOCK BETWEEN THIGHS · BLOCK UNDER SACRUM · STERNUM LIFT · PRESSING UPPER THIGHS

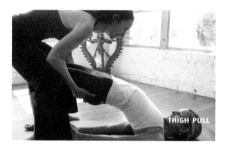
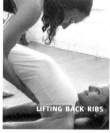
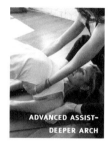
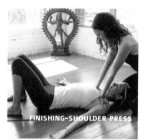

THIGH PULL · LIFTING BACK RIBS · ADVANCED ASSIST- DEEPER ARCH · FINISHING-SHOULDER PRESS

COMMON MISALIGNMENTS

- Feet and legs turned out, not parallel
- Lower back holding most of the arch, leading to compression and a crunched feeling
- Shoulders tight
- Chest collapsed, upper back body not activated

ASSISTS

Beginners: Set up a good starting position, feet hip-width and parallel. To keep parallel position, you can put a block in between or belt thighs, just above the knees. Help students maintain parallel position of legs to prevent compression in sacrum/lower back. Once feet are set, take a good look *from the side* and notice places where you might create extra space and expansion. Often, action stalls out in the legs, so pose looks flat from the side, pelvis dropped and/or chest collapsed. Put a block horizontally or vertically under sacrum to create more support underneath. Shift block from low to high to help find the right height. Chin moves toward the chest, weight centered on feet. To strengthen legs, you might place a block on top of pelvis and cue student to lift it UP.

Beginners/Intermediate: For tight shoulders, palms stay along sides of body, otherwise hands interlace underneath. Inner, upper arms rotate externally, from the inside out, to create opening across chest. I encourage students to scoot their shoulders all the way underneath the body, so that from above, the shoulders almost disappear. A light touch or press at the sternum encourages them to lift chest UP. You can also invite more lift and support to upper chest with a belt. Seated behind, slide belt just behind the shoulders and draw back on belt gently.

Intermediate: By the time students can hold pose steadily, look for a nice even arch, with active feet and legs. To strengthen legs and invite more lift in pelvis, from above, press firmly on outer, upper thighs as you cue student to press up against your hands. You'll see a visible lift in lower body. Alternately, you can reach underneath thigh creases—where thighs meet buttocks—and give a firm tug upward. And yet another nice assist: from above, reach underneath the upper back and hug upper back ribs close to where shoulder blades come together. Lift up slightly, then allow your hands to massage and slide toward middle back, tracing along either side of the spine, helping the surrounding muscles relax.

Advanced: This assist invites a deeper arch in middle to upper back. Without crowding in too close, sit behind with your feet braced sideways against shoulders. From here, reach underneath rib cage and gently lift up the middle back. You'll see the chest moving toward you during the assist. Keep that support going for a few breaths, so student can settle in. I often massage along either side of the spine, traveling my hands from *middle toward upper* back. The extra contact with your hands releases extra tension along the spine and feels fantastic.

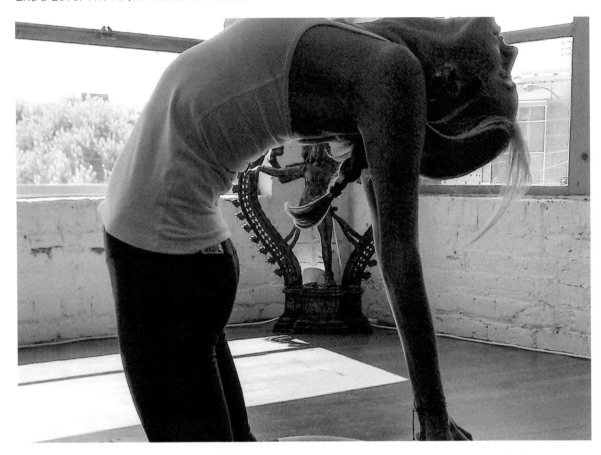

USTRASANA – CAMEL POSE

Camel Pose runs counter to all of our natural instincts. The front pelvis, lower trunk and psoas muscles are opened up, challenging our fight or flight reflex. Camel opens up the chest and shoulders, which tend to spend most of their day rounded forward over work, a computer screen or the wheel of our car. It opens up the heart, which instinctively wants to protect itself from emotional hurt, or the fear that the love we express won't be returned. For all these reasons, you would think Camel Pose would be impossible, but it's absolutely exhilarating once the right alignment comes into play.

A moderate to deep back bend, Camel can't be forced. As with Bridge Pose, students first have to anchor through the legs and pelvis with proper alignment, gradually inviting the upper back, chest and shoulders to open. This takes time and patience. Eventually, the energy and arc of the back bend moves through evenly, from tailbone to base of skull.

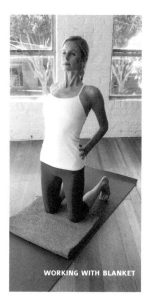

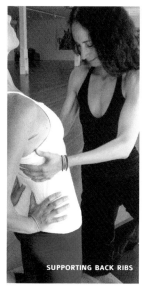

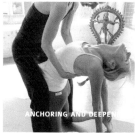

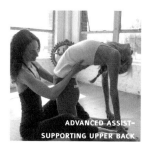

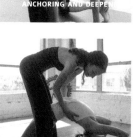

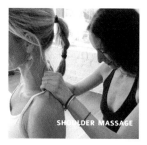

WORKING WITH BLANKET

SUPPORTING BACK RIBS

ANCHORING AND DEEPEN

ADVANCED ASSIST-
SUPPORTING UPPER BACK

BABY WHEEL

SHOULDER MASSAGE

COMMON MISALIGNMENTS

- Hips not aligned over knees, pelvis retracted back
- Chest or lower back collapsed
- Shoulders hunched

ASSISTS

Beginners: Use a folded blanket to pad knees at hip-width apart, legs parallel. For an easier reach, raise heels up, tucking toes under. Let student test out pose, starting with hands on sacrum, tipping upper chest back a little further each time. For the assist, simply anchor their hips with your hands, then with a light touch or press point, encourage a lift UP in the sternum. You can also support the student, as you reach around back ribs with your hands, as student tries lowering hands or fingertips to heels, one hand at a time, or both together. Keep bracing hips and/or back ribs as they settle into pose. Make sure hips stay over knees, tailbone down, with no collapsing or hinging in lower back. Help them lift up after last breath count by supporting hips or back ribs.

Beginners/Intermediate: Once beginners can come into pose more fully, have them keep chin to chest and work on lifting the sternum with deep, steady breathing. Head stays in line with shoulders instead of just "falling back."

Intermediate: For students with good lower body alignment, anchor the pose and deepen the arch. Stand in front and secure their hips with your legs, then reach around back ribs to give a lift up from underneath. You'll see the chest lifting. Watch for compression in neck; if extended too far back, the position feels uncomfortable, inhibits breathing and chokes off the pose. If this happens, ask student to lift chin to chest, holding a strong open shape with the neck in *neutral* position. Let the neck extend and head go back only if chest is lifted, upper body is relaxed and open and breath is steady.

Advanced: Sitting in front, stretch your legs around theirs, resting your feet on their calves. With their legs anchored, use your hands to give support at upper back thigh crease and around back ribs, expressly working to deepen the arch in *middle* to *upper* back, legs and pelvis keeping strong alignment. Watch the front body and see that the chest lifts strongly. Hips shouldn't hinge backwards, but stay just above knees.

For Baby Wheel Pose, you'll also anchor the base as the chest opens. Stand in front, anchoring outer thighs with your feet. Reach underneath their body to lift and support back ribs, drawing back of heart up. A light touch to the sternum also works great here to help bring attention and lift in upper chest. Students love a shoulder massage when they come out of a pose.

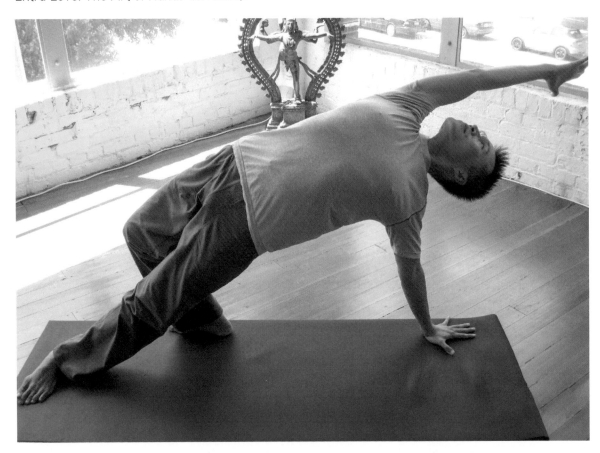

WILD THING INTO THREE-QUARTER WHEEL

You make my heart sing! The Troggs from England made this song a number one hit in 1966. Jimi Hendrix re-invented the song while lighting his guitar on fire at the 1967 Monterey Pop Festival.

Wild Thing is a popular and fun pose that feels great, develops arm strength and helps students experience a moderate back bend from the simplicity of Downward Facing Dog or Plank Pose. In an advanced variation, it builds toward Three-Quarter Wheel Pose or Full Wheel Pose. The best assist for Wild Thing is helping students find the right foot/hand pattern. Without it, the foundation gets weak and they miss out on the fun. From a secure base, you can easily lift the student way up, so they feel like they're flying. You make everything groovy!

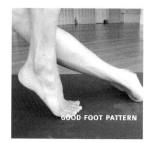
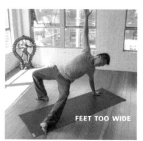
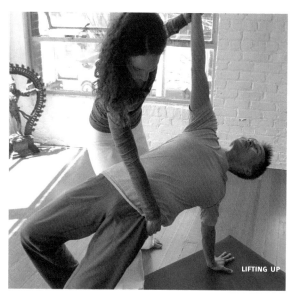
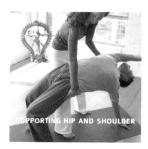
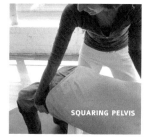

GOOD FOOT PATTERN

FEET TOO WIDE

SUPPORTING HIP AND SHOULDER

SQUARING PELVIS

LIFTING UP

COMMON MISALIGNMENTS

- Feet splayed apart
- Bottom hand too far forward, creating shoulder instability

ASSISTS

Beginners: First, set up foot pattern. Starting in Plank Pose, student steps back foot just behind opposite calf (legs almost touching) with bent knee aligned directly above ankle. The supporting leg, fully extended, turns out so edge of foot rests on floor. For hand pattern, supporting wrist (of lower arm) is directly below supporting shoulder, as in Side Plank Pose. You often see supporting hand too far forward, stressing the elbow or shoulder joint. To assist from here, stand *behind* and facing in and reach one hand around bottom hip, also taking top wrist. Lift straight UP from underneath as you also lift and extend top arm. Feels great!

Intermediate: From Downward Facing Dog, with one leg up, knee bent and hip open, the student steps underneath into a bigger version of Wild Thing. Feet are wider here, building toward Three-Quarter Wheel. Before student settles into pose, if the feet are too far apart, help square the feet *hip-width apart* and parallel, ankles directly under bent knees. Pelvis also squares off, facing upward. If supporting hand is too far forward on mat, have student shift the whole position forward, until supporting shoulder aligns over bottom wrist. For the assist, stand in same position as above, reach under back thigh crease, where thigh meets the buttock and take top wrist. Lift straight up from underneath as you extend top arm. Cue a lift/ expansion of whole front body equally, from front thighs to upper chest. You'd be surprised how much lift you create with this simple action, once feet are in the right position. So groovy!

Advanced: Assist progression from Three-Quarter Wheel into Full Wheel (Urdhva Dhanurasana). Start with previous assists, support upper back moving toward Wheel, then help set the hand underneath in good alignment, feet parallel, for Wheel. Help flip it back over, gliding through good alignment, working back to Downward Facing Dog.

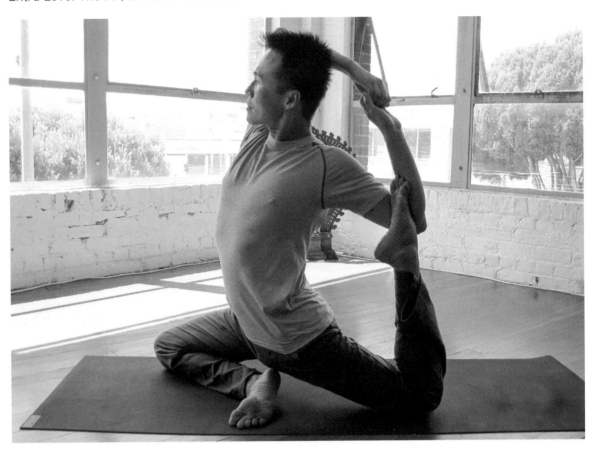

MERMAID AND EKA PADA RAJA KAPOTASANA — KING PIGEON

Mermaid and King Pigeon are beautiful positions, originating in Pigeon Pose (I covered assists to Pigeon in *Extra Love: Volume 1* and repeat many tips here). Both are deep back bends, suitable for intermediate to advanced students, where the thighs, buttocks and deep pelvic muscles provide a strong foundation. The spine, hips and shoulders also must be very flexible. Your goal in assisting is to stabilize the whole shape so students ready for these poses can go deeper.

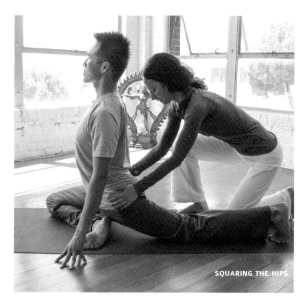

SQUARING THE HIPS

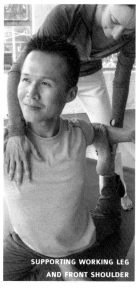

SUPPORTING WORKING LEG
AND FRONT SHOULDER

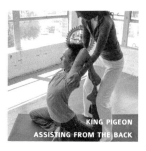

KING PIGEON
ASSISTING FROM THE BACK

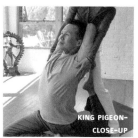

KING PIGEON-
CLOSE-UP

COMMON MISALIGNMENTS

- Front foot too far away from pelvis
- Back leg lacks stretch in quadriceps, difficult to bend knee and square off pelvis
- Pose swings open to the side or lower back compresses

ASSISTS

Intermediate: As you would for Pigeon, set up a stable base by adjusting front foot close enough so that student feels anchored in their seat. Starting with the front foot too far forward puts more pressure on front knee or hip, tilting the pelvis and making the pose more difficult. Pelvis and chest should face directly forward. Align back leg so that top of thigh/knee/shin and foot are all centered on floor. Standing behind, help to square off the hips as you would for Pigeon and support back ribs so the student lifts up evenly through both sides of body and avoids compressing lower back. The position should feel square and lifted.

Once student is ready to bend back knee to take foot, kneel at the side or front. Create a lift *up* the front body to prevent sagging in lower abdomen or lower back and bring attention to *uddiyana bandha*. I often place a fingertip there and tell student to lift *up*. Using both hands, you can also come around and again lift up back ribs. These are similar assists to Warrior 1 and in fact the torso position aims for the same basic shape. Look for an even stretch across front of chest and shoulders and an even lift through sides of body.

Intermediate/Advanced: Moving around to working leg, help student keep a secure grip on foot, or hook foot inside elbow (for Mermaid). If this is as far as they want to go, kneel down next to working leg and stabilize it with your hip or hand. Reach around the back with your opposite hand and stabilize opposite upper shoulder/upper chest. Solidly anchor the two points, as student breathes deep and works toward a fuller back bend. I usually hold this assist until the last breath count, then ease off carefully.

Advanced: For Eka Pada Raja Kapotasana, create a stable base/lift up front body as in Mermaid. Once student has the foot, your assists are similar. I usually assist from the side or back and help to brace both ends, where feet meet hands, counterbalanced by upper front body. My favorite place to assist is from the back, standing or kneeling close in, where I can support several places at once—back leg, elbow position and shoulders. Supported all around, students can breathe deep, open the chest and settle into a nice, full position.

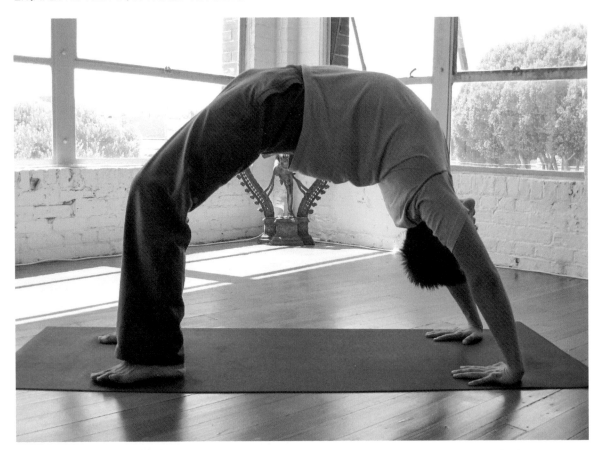

URDHVA DHANURASANA – UPWARD FACING BOW/FULL WHEEL POSE

Urdhva Dhanurasana is a deep back bend, very challenging for beginners and even intermediate students. The great teacher Dharma Mittra says that difficulty in this pose comes from lack of faith, referring to the pose's meaning, from the Sanskrit root *dhan* = to offer up to God or the divine. It does take tremendous faith, to lie on a sweaty mat, place your hands behind your ears, press down with hands and feet, lift your abdomen and heart straight up toward the sky, hang your head upside down, arch the entire spine evenly.... *and* breathe! Dharma calls this pose an act of adoration to the Lord and his advice inspires me every time.

Wheel Pose combines success factors from all other back bends: strong, parallel legs and feet, ample stretch across the quadriceps, strength through pelvis, even flexibility through the whole spine, open chest and shoulders and strong, well-aligned arms to help complete the circle. Intimate familiarity with the pose helps you assist students confidently and effectively. This is a pose you have to know in your own body, inside and out and how to make it work under different conditions. For all levels, your goal is to encourage the essential shape of the pose, with an even arch, equal weight distribution and an experience for the student that's free of struggle or difficulty.

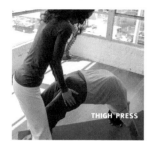
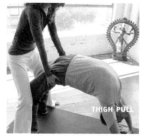
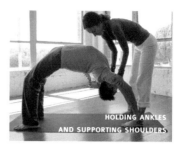
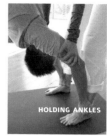

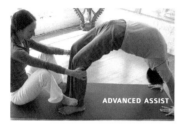
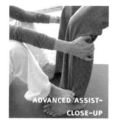
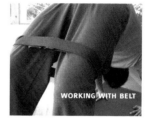
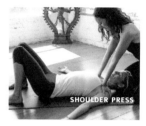

COMMON MISALIGNMENTS

- Feet and legs out of parallel position
- Uneven curvature through back
- Uneven weight distribution from feet to hands
- Arms can't extend due to tight shoulders

ASSISTS

Beginners: Start in Half-Wheel Pose, with the same alignment and assists. Feet/legs parallel. You can belt thighs (just above knees), or place a block between thighs, to keep hip-width alignment of feet. Once feet are set, take a good look *from the side*, as you would for Half Wheel and notice places where you might create space and expansion. Often, action stalls out in the legs, so pose looks flat from the side, pelvis dropped or chest collapsed. Put a block under sacrum for added support and space underneath. Chest moves up toward chin. Read through the beginners' assists for Half Wheel and repeat them here.

Intermediate: To develop stronger legs and more lift in pelvis, from above, press firmly on outer top thighs as student pushes up against your hands. This assist usually initiates a visible lift. You can also reach underneath and give a firm lift under the back thigh creases, just where thighs meet buttocks, giving a slight inner spiral action to outer thighs. To support the arms, standing behind, reach underneath and cup your hands under the shoulders as you gently lift up. This helps pull the arch further up the spine. As you do this, straddle the arms with your legs, helping to bring the wrists, elbows and shoulders into alignment. Look for even weight distribution from feet to hands.

Some students, usually men, have the strength to lift up, but can't extend the arms due to tight shoulders. Then, you have to create more space through the arms. Stand behind, about 8 to 10 inches. Have student firmly hold your ankles. Help draw their elbows inward, to set shoulders on upper back. As they push up into Wheel, extending their arms, reach underneath, cup your hands under the shoulders and lift up. If their elbows start to swing open, straddle their arms with your legs, to bring wrists, elbows and shoulders into alignment. Keep your hands under shoulders as they hold your ankles. Look for active feet and legs, weight distribution even between hands and feet. *Ease them back down after last breath count.* Your stance is knees bent, using *mula bandha*.

Advanced: For students with a very strong pose, challenge the legs with an assist similar to Camel. Sit down in front and anchor their feet in place with yours. Hold just below knee crease, around back of upper calf muscles and firmly pull their legs toward you. You're leaning back slightly, creating a resistance point. From here, encourage them to "straighten" their legs. The assist creates a push/pull sensation, strengthens the legs and—for very flexible yogis—helps evenly distribute the back bend throughout spine.

All levels: Once student releases pose, resting on their back, press their shoulders down, leaning in with a bit of your body weight.

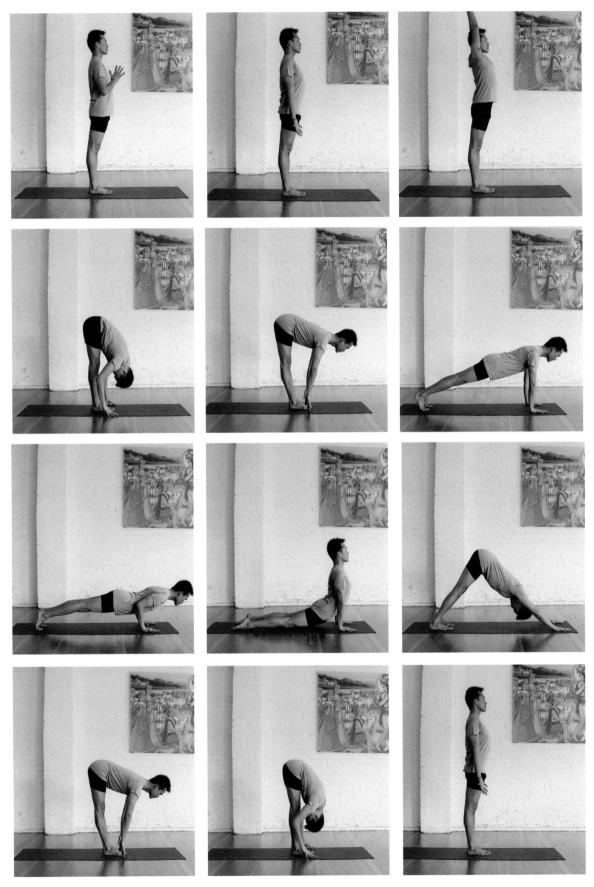

SURYA NAMASKAR – SUN SALUTATIONS

It takes real finesse to assist Sun Salutations gracefully and effectively. Since students are in constant motion, you have to be very much in the moment and with them every step of the way. Knowing the poses and transitions inside and out helps you anticipate the right assists, not only in Surya Namaskar, but also in other *vinyasa* (flowing) sequences. This is the time to pull together all your skills from assisting the individual poses and add to that a good sense of timing and rhythm.

The Guiding Principles highlighted the importance of varying your approach—advice that applies here. For every pose and transition within Surya Namaskar, you have several assisting options. There isn't just one assist for Mountain Pose, followed by another for Standing Forward Bend and so on. Instead, you should carefully observe how the student moves and individualize your approach according to what he or she presents. The beauty of this process is that it's entirely customized to the student. Your own approach depends upon the alignment and technical refinements you want to facilitate for each student's body, the way you want to direct energy and breath in each pose and your student's level of experience, strength and flexibility on any given day. Learn and practice one or two basic assists for each pose, then weave in other assists tailored to your students' needs.

Once you are comfortable assisting Surya Namaskar, concentrate on one student at a time, staying with them for at least one entire cycle. In my experience, this is more effective and powerful than moving down a row of mats, trying to reach many students quickly. Rather than an "assembly line" approach, think of customizing your assists. The student will feel more warmed up, your assists helping them connect more deeply to their body and breath as their practice begins. They will feel this connection throughout the class.

The first section takes you through Surya Namaskar, pose by pose, highlighting major misalignments as well as the *most* effective assists to use while students are in motion. Assists in this section are focused on misalignments instead of being organized according to the experience level of the student and most are great for beginners. If the assist is better suited to an intermediate or advanced student, I'll mention it in the description. Every assist allows for an interval of approximately one inhale or one exhale.

The second, shorter section illustrates several different assisting variations for Surya Namaskar.

Ready, set... let's go greet the sun!

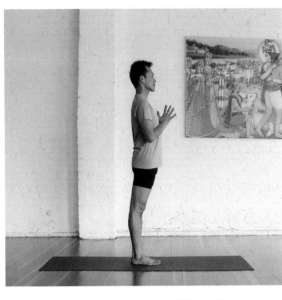

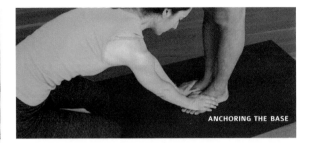
ANCHORING THE BASE

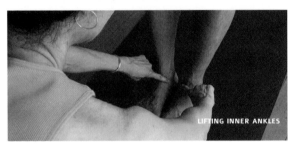
LIFTING INNER ANKLES

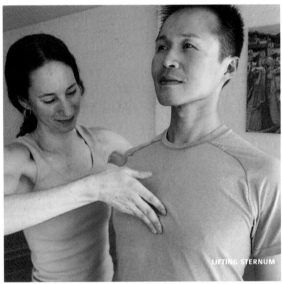
LIFTING STERNUM

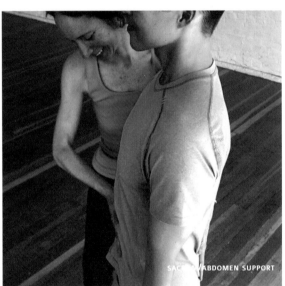
SACRUM/ABDOMEN SUPPORT

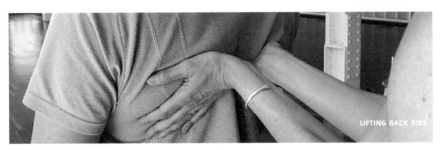
LIFTING BACK RIBS

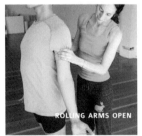
ROLLING ARMS OPEN

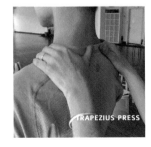
TRAPEZIUS PRESS

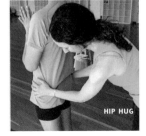
HIP HUG

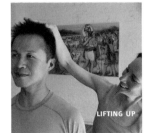
LIFTING UP

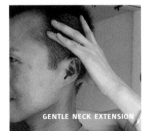
GENTLE NECK EXTENSION

TADASANA – MOUNTAIN POSE

We looked at Mountain Pose in depth in the earlier section on standing poses. Within each round of Surya Namaskar you have two chances to enhance Mountain Pose: at the beginning, when the student is ready to start the cycle and at the end of a round, when the student is more warmed up and holding for an extra breath or two. I use many of these assists interchangeably, depending on what I see, repeating some to reinforce important alignment or form.

COMMON MISALIGNMENTS
- Weak base—feet not active/inner ankles collapsed
- Slouching or swayback
- Shoulders rounded, chest dropped, general lack of confidence
- Pose needs more lift *up* front of body

ASSISTS

To activate feet/ankles: Get down low, spread out toes and even out weight on both feet. Press feet down with your hands and cue student to lift up through body from the feet. Bring attention to inner ankles, swiping your fingertips upward and suggesting a "lift."

For slouching/swayback: Slouching/swayback are common in Mountain Pose and can suggest anything from basic hesitation or lack of confidence to weakness in spine or core abdominal muscles. Standing to the side, correct sagging in lower back or abdomen by placing one hand flat on sacrum, other hand flat on lower abdomen. Tailbone lengthens down without tucking, as lower abdomen lifts up strongly. You should see a visible lift. If not, tell student to lift lower abdomen in and up while also lifting the chest. Side waists should lengthen.

For collapsed chest: Correct slouching/swayback first. Then standing to side, use a light touch at sternum and cue student to lift up against your touch. If you're standing behind, gently hug and lift the back ribs to elongate the back body and create a lift in front chest. For rounded shoulders, stand behind and, holding the biceps, roll open upper, inner arms. This assist helps spread collarbones and lift chest.

For more lift/length through side body: Stand behind. Hug and anchor the hips firmly *downward* with your hands, creating a grounding point from which student can lift up along both sides of body. Great for all students, especially intermediate/advanced.

To create more confidence/lift up through body: Put a hand flat on top of head and encourage student to lift from the feet *all the way up* (this is a fun assist to do with partners, outside of Surya Namaskar, using blocks). Or place your thumbs on the underside/occipital ridge of skull, with fingers lightly spread and placed around sides of head. Keep your hands steady and with a light to moderate touch, lift up *gently* to encourage extension.

To ground student into pose: Massage/press down trapezius muscles as a reminder to release/soften the upper shoulders. After a few cycles of Surya Namaskar, students really love this assist.

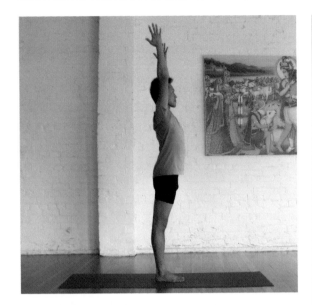

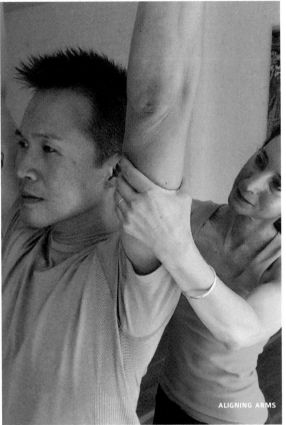

ALIGNING ARMS

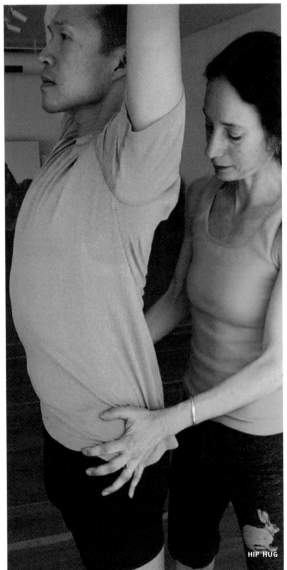

HIP HUG

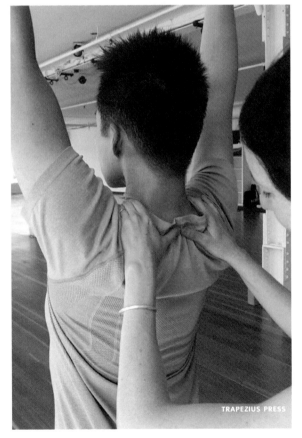

TRAPEZIUS PRESS

URDHVA HASTASANA — ARMS OVERHEAD

Forward momentum in Surya Namaskar comes from Urdhva Hastasana, arms reaching symbolically overhead in a moment of fullness and abundance. Pay close attention to the position, because it forecasts other assists and tweaks to related poses (e.g., High Lunge, Warrior 1, Handstand) you might need to use later in class.

COMMON MISALIGNMENTS

- Swayback with ribs out
- Arms too far back
- Shoulders lifted

ASSISTS

For swayback: Use the "hip hug and anchor" assist from Mountain Pose to prevent arching in lower back as arms lift overhead. Swayback is common among beginners as well as flexible, advanced students, who like to hyper-extend. Hyper-extension here is often seen in Downward Facing Dog, as well.

To correct arms: Except among very strong students, the lower back tends to collapse when arms reach too far behind head. Realign arms alongside/just in front of ears and roll the inner, upper arms open from the inside out (as in Tadasana). Holding the biceps, rotate upper arms so palms spin to face in toward center. Assist just as arms arrive overhead, so student incorporates the feeling and alignment with the actual movement.

For hunched shoulders: An ingrained habit, usually. Firmly press trapezius muscles down. Repeat as needed.

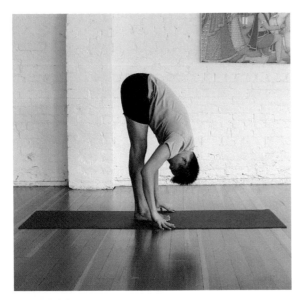

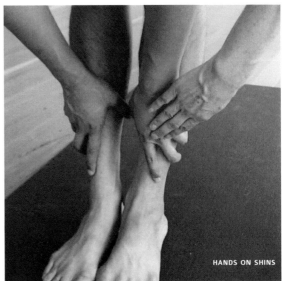

HANDS ON SHINS

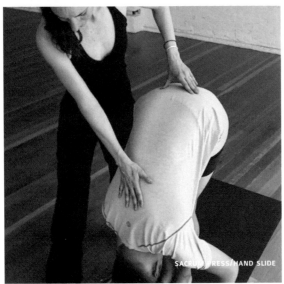

SACRUM PRESS/HAND SLIDE

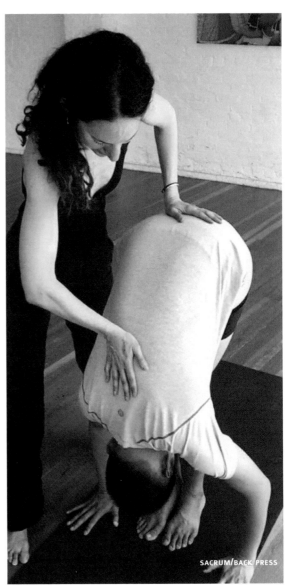

SACRUM/BACK PRESS

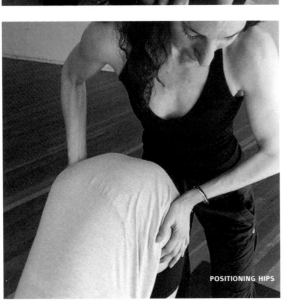

POSITIONING HIPS

UTTANASANA – STANDING FORWARD BEND

Extra Love: Volume 1 covered Uttanasana in the section on Forward Bends. I deconstructed the pose and gave options for assisting and modifying when holding for several breaths. When moving within Surya Namaskar, the pose is easier for most students; you might see just a few common misalignments and other issues. The gesture of bowing down is quite beautiful; try to facilitate as much ease and fluidity as possible.

COMMON MISALIGNMENTS

- Tight hamstrings and rounded back
- Weight pushed forward or backward on feet (unsteady foundation)
- Shoulders/neck hunched

ASSISTS

For tight hamstrings: Right away, have student place hands on shins or thighs when they come forward, instead of trying to reach floor, or position two blocks near the hands, to raise floor up as student comes forward. Knees can soften or bend, if needed.

For rounded back: For beginners, slide or place your hand on back to encourage length and relaxation, just as or after they come forward. For intermediate/advanced students, stand to the side, with a foot wedged sideways against student's heels. Place one hand flat on sacrum, pressing down firmly and slide other hand down rounded part of back to encourage length. The action: rooting down into the legs, while lengthening spine. Your action dovetails with the exhale into the pose.

To deepen fold: After several rounds or a thorough warm-up in Surya Namaskar, work to deepen the fold. Same as assist above: stand to the side, with foot wedged sideways against student's heels. Place one hand flat on sacrum, pressing down firmly; slide other hand down rounded part of back for length. The action: rooting down into the legs, while lengthening spine. Your action dovetails with the exhale.

For uneven weight on feet: Viewed from above or the side, you can tell if weight in Uttanasana is pushed forward (toes gripping) or backward (sitting backward into heels, backs of knees or legs pushing backwards). Just after student comes into the pose, quickly reposition their hips so weight is centered and even on feet. Back of hips should align directly above heels.

For shoulder tension: After the exhale into Uttanasana, reach over and quickly massage tension from neck, trapezius muscles or shoulders.

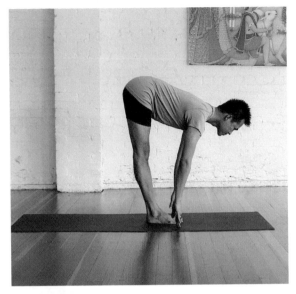

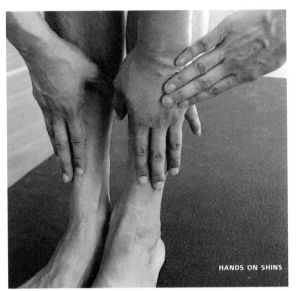

HANDS ON SHINS

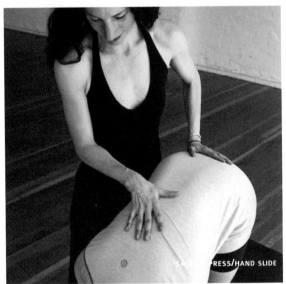

SACRUM PRESS/HAND SLIDE

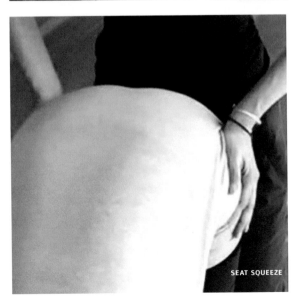

SEAT SQUEEZE

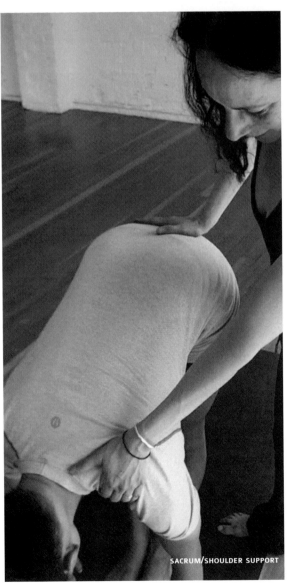

SACRUM/SHOULDER SUPPORT

FLAT BACK – PREPARATION FOR LUNGE, PLANK OR CHATURANGA

In this transition, the student lengthens the upper body in anticipation of the next position—either Chaturanga, Plank or Lunge Pose. Though tight hamstrings might prevent fullest extension of the spine, you can easily assist the position toward a nice, flat back—an ideal setup for Chaturanga, where the chest actually comes slightly forward as the legs/feet go back.

COMMON MISALIGNMENTS

- Back rounded
- Shoulders hunched

ASSISTS

For rounded back: If student can't reach floor here (or in Uttanasana), quickly position their hands to rest on their shins, so they can comfortably lengthen the torso forward on the inhale, creating a nice, flat back. Slight bend in knees is also fine.

To get more extension in back: As student lengthens forward, anchor one hand flat on the sacrum and slide other hand *down* the back, toward sacrum, just as the inhale finishes up. The feeling of your hand sliding down their back encourages them to lengthen forward. Release the assist before the exhale back into Plank/Chaturanga.

For more extension: I call this the Seat Squeeze. Standing behind, hug the outer hips/buttocks firmly in toward center, drawing the hips back ever so slightly. Create a little resistance from the back, as student extends forward on the inhale. Quickly step away before the exhale into next position. Good for intermediate/advanced students.

For hunched shoulders: Stand to side, root down slightly on sacrum with one hand and with opposite hand, lengthen chest out, holding just underneath shoulder. Synchronize your assist on the inhale, as student prepares. This assist gives student a feeling of extending forward, without lifting or tensing shoulders.

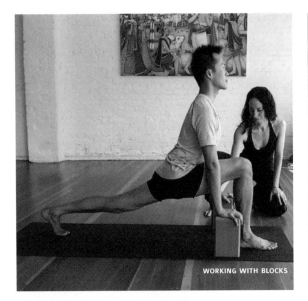

WORKING WITH BLOCKS

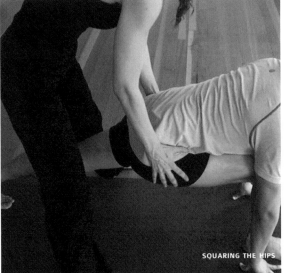

SQUARING THE HIPS

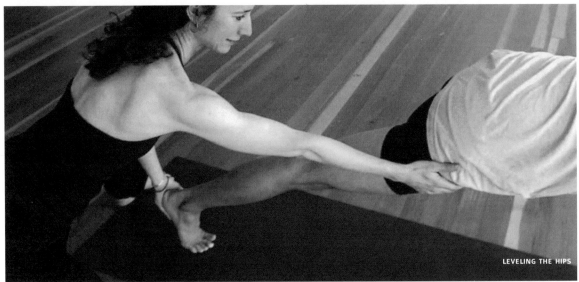

LEVELING THE HIPS

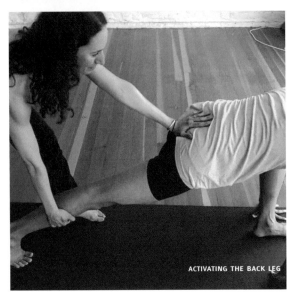

ACTIVATING THE BACK LEG

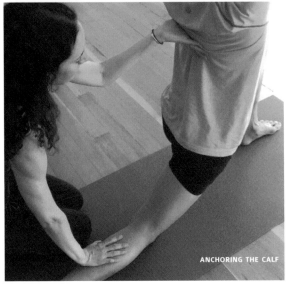

ANCHORING THE CALF

LUNGE POSE

Many versions of Surya Namaskar call for lunging forward and back, with back knee on or off the floor, in transition between poses. Front knee alignment, level hips and full extension through back leg are important elements. I assist Lunge Pose often, because the simple, lunging action suggests a student's approach to more intense poses, including High Lunge, Warrior 1 and Rotated Side Angle Pose. The front and back legs have to work well together.

COMMON MISALIGNMENTS

- Front knee misaligned
- Hips/sacrum tilted
- Back leg needs more power

ASSISTS

For front knee alignment: For regular Lunge Pose, make sure front, bent knee aligns directly over ankle, with shin perpendicular to floor. In Low Lunge, front knee can come forward a bit, but stays in parallel alignment and extends no further than toes. Beginners can have two blocks at their hands to use for stepping forward and back.

For tilted hips: A common misalignment, even for advanced students, so here are a few options. Standing behind, brace and help square hips to front just as student arrives into the lunge. Or, standing to the side or behind, you can lift the lower, sagging hip to level it off with the higher hip. At the same time, support opposite back leg, shin or heel. The assist integrates the feeling of level hips and strong back leg. Finally, make sure feet don't over-cross when stepping forward/back into Lunge Pose, which tends to tilt hips further. Sacrum stays level and stable.

To activate back leg: Place one hand firmly on sacrum, bracing it forward slightly. At the same time, hold underneath back thigh or shin, lifting and pulling back slightly. Student feels a nice push/pull between the two points as back leg awakens.

To expand upper body in Low Lunge: Anchor the base (back foot or calf), then step in to lift back ribs just behind the heart. You can also put one hand behind the heart, lifting up, as you take forearms to lift and support upper chest. A fingertip on the sternum helps lift upper chest and another just below the navel, at *uddiyana bandha*, helps lift and support lower abdomen. Try to prevent advanced students from sitting into the lower back.

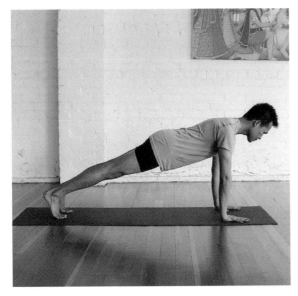

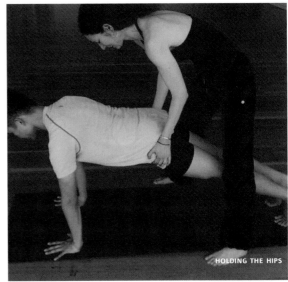

HOLDING THE HIPS

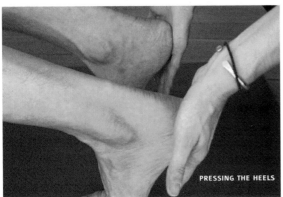

PRESSING THE HEELS

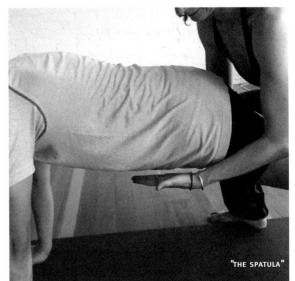

"THE SPATULA"

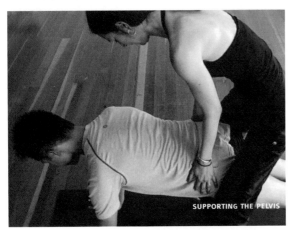

SUPPORTING THE PELVIS

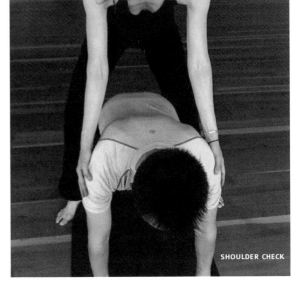

SHOULDER CHECK

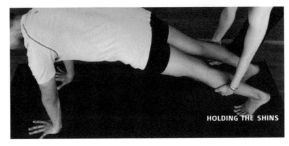

HOLDING THE SHINS

PLANK POSE

The strength we develop in Plank Pose carries into Chaturanga, Upward and Downward Dog, Side Plank, Handstand and many other poses. Plank teaches us how to hold the body's weight up in space, while maintaining lightness and moving seamlessly through Surya Namaskar. Many students benefit from assists and refinements to Plank, including beginners or anyone brand new to yoga, as well as women just building arm strength and continuing students needing small tweaks to alignment or form.

COMMON MISALIGNMENTS

- Legs not carrying strength of pose
- Pelvis or lower back dropped, or pelvis too high
- Not enough strength in arms to hold parallel position
- Neck unsupported, head dropped

ASSISTS

To support and strengthen legs: In Plank, both ends (arms and legs) each carry about fifty percent of the pose's strength. There should be even weight distribution between the hands and feet. This is easier said than done. If the back end is giving out and legs look visibly weak (but upper body looks steady), hold underneath shins or thighs to provide support. To further activate and strengthen legs, stand behind and have student press heels straight back into your hands. For a held Plank (not within the flow of Surya Namaskar), have student squeeze a block between the thighs. All these assists—in fact, *any* contact with the legs or feet—increases sensation and awareness of lower body in Plank Pose.

To support pelvis and legs (option 1): For many students, women especially, the pelvis (as the center of gravity) feels like the heaviest point. To assist, hold hips securely, keeping them parallel to floor as student comes into Plank. From here, maintain the hold as they lower into Chaturanga or variations. If the pelvis happens to be lifted up higher than rest of body, bring hips in line. If holding Plank for a few breaths, stand above the student with your feet turned out and knees bent and straddle the upper thighs just between your calves, supporting the pelvis in position parallel to the floor. Transfer your hands to their hips just before the exhale into Chaturanga.

To support pelvis and legs (option 2): Make a double "Spatula" with your hands, palms flat and facing up and place them just underneath hips as the student comes into Plank. This assist cues lower abdominals to lift in and up (*uddiyana bandha*) and prevents sagging through the pelvis. *Keep the Spatula assist as they lower into Chaturanga.*

For arm/shoulder alignment: I usually do a visual or manual shoulder check to make sure shoulders are aligned over wrists, with arms well extended but not rigid. If student isn't ready to hold plank (the legs, pelvis, back, chest or arms are collapsing) have them put the knees down and work with Half Chaturanga until the arms get stronger.

To support the neck: Encourage beginners and even strong intermediate/advanced students to hold neck in line with spine, supporting weight of the head. Gaze is slightly forward, chin slightly lifted.

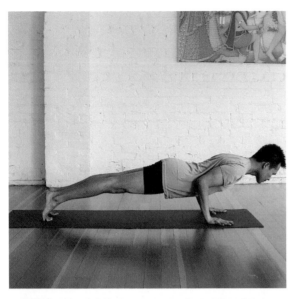

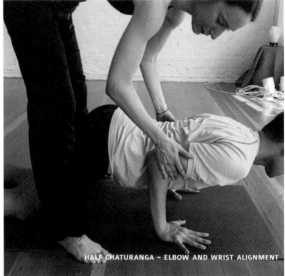

HALF CHATURANGA – ELBOW AND WRIST ALIGNMENT

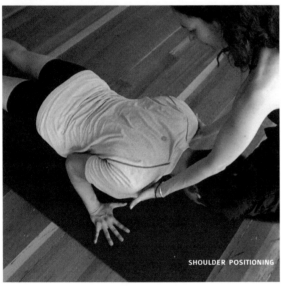

SHOULDER POSITIONING

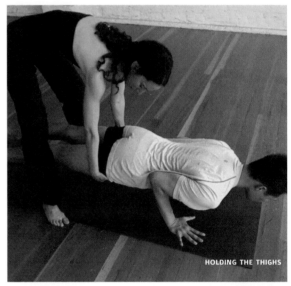

HOLDING THE THIGHS

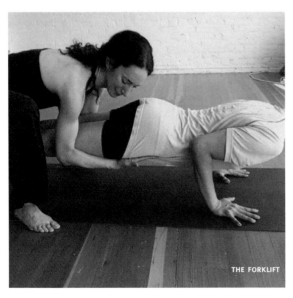

THE FORKLIFT

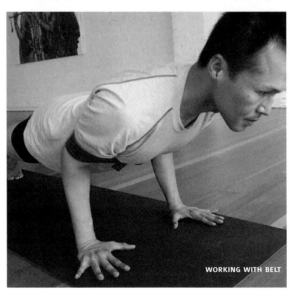

WORKING WITH BELT

CHATURANGA DANDASANA – FOUR-LIMBED STAFF POSE

Chaturanga builds strength, heat and power—Yoga's equivalent to the push-up. Easily the most challenging Surya Namaskar position, Chaturanga alignment is difficult for students to develop, simply because the pose is so hard to hold for more than a moment or two. Like Plank Pose, the challenge here is teaching use of the whole body to stay up—keeping legs, torso, chest and chin parallel to floor. Students should feel equal length through body, applying effort to extend forward through the upper body as lower body draws back. Ideally, the pose doesn't feel "heavy," but instead moves seamlessly between Plank and Up Dog.

COMMON MISALIGNMENTS

- Hands too far forward or back
- Elbows open to side, shoulders up
- Shoulders too close to floor
- Pelvis dropped toward floor, or raised up

ASSISTS

For hand position: Correct form in Plank Pose—shoulders over wrists—gets students off to a good start. As elbows bend straight back, they stay over wrists. Observe hands, arms and shoulders and help maintain elbow/wrist alignment. Torso stays parallel to floor, chest comes slightly forward, roughly same distance from floor as knees. Chin lifts slightly, gaze is forward. Work one-on-one with beginners to break down the pose, review alignment and build confidence. Teach Half Chaturanga as an alternative until students are ready for full pose.

For wide elbows/lifted shoulders: This is a common misalignment and usually signals lack of arm strength. To assist, step around and help draw elbows straight back, at the same time encouraging student to draw shoulder blades down the back, chest moving forward. You may have to reposition elbows several times before students get the hang of it. If they're still struggling, use Half Chaturanga. For men with very muscular biceps (who have trouble bending elbows straight back), set hands slightly further apart at the start of Plank Pose.

For dropped shoulders: Many students lower shoulders too far forward, bending the elbows too much on the descent into pose, which can strain the upper body. Among advanced students, I've observed a strong correlation between dropped shoulders and lower back injury—a further reason to watch and assist carefully. Elbows in Chaturanga bend far less than students think—no more than ninety degrees, with shoulders staying in same line as torso, pelvis and legs. For me personally, anything more than a two-inch elbow bend means I "bottom out." From the back, side or front, help guide position of shoulders, indicating at what level they're too low, or just right.

For dropped pelvis or weak legs: Call in your reinforcements from Plank Pose! To support pelvis, hold hips on descent to Chaturanga, or continue the Spatula assist. To support legs/lower body, hold underneath thighs or shins, or try the Forklift. Stand above with your knees bent, elbows bent at ninety degrees. Place your forearms just underneath student's thighs, as they prepare to lower from Plank to Chaturanga, your fingertips resting on the front of their hips. Keep your arms in this position. Like a forklift, steady them as they lower down. Go for correct, lower body alignment: pelvis/legs parallel to floor, knees straight, tailbone/pubic bone move toward each other slightly (i.e., *mula bandha* activated), lower abdominals lifting in and up to support weight of pelvis. If pelvis tilts up, reposition it parallel to floor, as in Plank.

Other assists for new students: Two props—a belt and a block—help new students playfully experiment with Chaturanga. Belt arms just above elbows. Have student practice holding pose with arms securely belted as chest extends forward. To support or activate legs, put a block just under or between thighs.

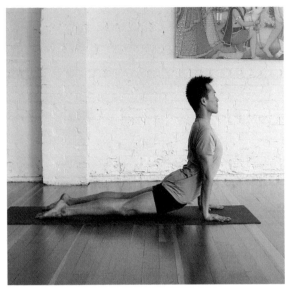

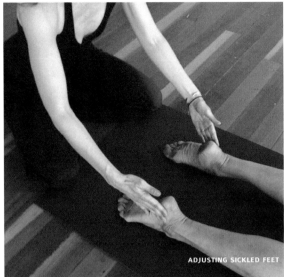

ADJUSTING SICKLED FEET

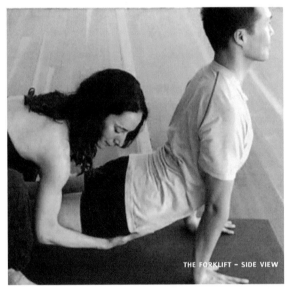

THE FORKLIFT – SIDE VIEW

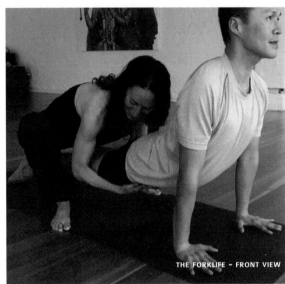

THE FORKLIFE – FRONT VIEW

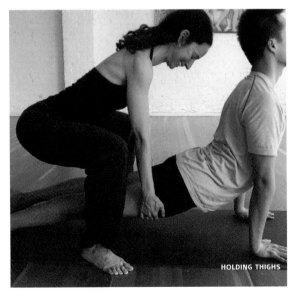

HOLDING THIGHS

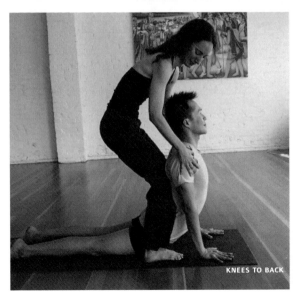

KNEES TO BACK

URDHVA MUKHA SVANASANA – UPWARD FACING DOG

Upward Facing Dog is a shining moment in Surya Namaskar! Done well, it's glorious, but done poorly—or confused with Cobra Pose—it can pinch the lower back and is no fun. Careful assists glide students into the right position, with attention to the entire body: legs, pelvis, torso, chest and arms. Movements leading up to this pose (Plank, Chaturanga) are important, too; assisting them well sets up the right conditions for Up Dog.

COMMON MISALIGNMENTS

- Feet sickled, taking strength out of legs
- Pelvis or thighs dropped, compressing lower back
- Shoulders lifted

ASSISTS

For sickled feet: Though a minor misalignment, I always correct sickled feet (meaning that they are turned in or out), because they can cause weakness in the legs, outer ankles and even the lower back. Lower legs must be very strong and aligned, since they hold up the whole back end of the pose. For internal sickling (heels collapsing outward—more common), rotate heels inward in line with back of knees. For external sickling (heels collapsing inward), rotate heels outward. Tops of feet should rest squarely on floor, hip-width apart and pointing straight back, toes spread.

For dropped pelvis: When the pelvis drops, you know that legs have lost parallel position to floor. To assist, catch underneath quadriceps as student lowers from Chaturanga. Coming into Up Dog, lift up slightly at same spot, supporting thighs, aiming to keep upper legs exactly parallel to floor. This takes pressure off legs so student can push firmly into floor, activating arms while bringing chest forward and up. Another option: continue the Forklift assist from Chaturanga. As student moves into Up Dog, keep your arms in same position, gliding them forward, supporting under thighs.

For lifted shoulders: Showing students the difference between Cobra and Upward Facing Dog, as well as working on arm strength (practicing Plank/Chaturanga and variations), are the best ways to prevent shoulder tension in Upward Facing Dog. I've noticed that strong, advanced students rarely lift shoulders in Up Dog. Among beginners, it's very common. The alternative, for them, is Cobra Pose, until arms can manage a steady, aligned ascent into Up Dog.

For chest expansion: For intermediate/advanced students, step in from behind with your feet turned in, knees bent slightly and aimed at bottom tips of student's shoulder blades. As student lifts up into pose, brace upper back with your knees and reach around to draw the shoulders open and wide with your hands—as if widening the collar bones—in one smooth, coordinated action. The action anchors the back, while lifting and opening the chest and upper back. This is a dynamic assist synchronized with student's movement on the inhale.

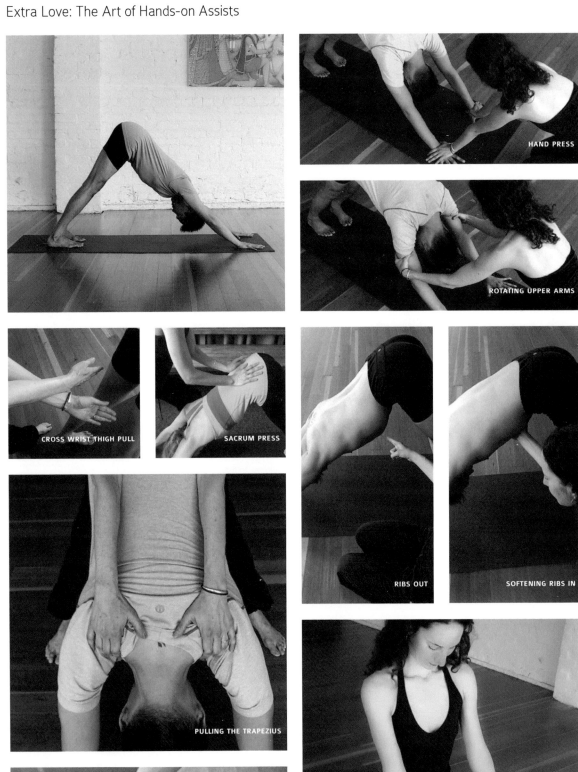

HAND PRESS

ROTATING UPPER ARMS

CROSS WRIST THIGH PULL

SACRUM PRESS

RIBS OUT

SOFTENING RIBS IN

PULLING THE TRAPEZIUS

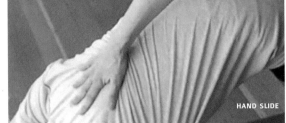

HAND SLIDE

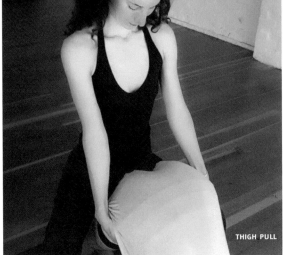

THIGH PULL

ADHO MUKHA SVANASANA – DOWNWARD FACING DOG

Downward Facing Dog is truly the working dog of Hatha Yoga. It awakens all the limbs, develops our ability to evenly distribute weight from front to back and right to left and teaches interrelation of all parts of the body to a unified whole. Students might spend five, ten or fifteen breaths in Down Dog, *multiple* times, within a typical *vinyasa* class. In some classes I think I've probably held Down Dogs for a cumulative half hour, sometimes working the pose itself and sometimes resting in the pose in between standing sequences.

Students' expressions of Down Dog will be as unique as their bodies. There is no universal or perfect assist for the pose. Instead, you have a marvelous opportunity to analyze what you see and apply your knowledge of how the pose can be optimized. Teachers often don't know how to adjust for restrictions such as tight hamstrings, stiff shoulders or hyper-flexibility. From many possibilities, the assists I describe here work well with Surya Namaskar, address the most common issues and give you a good foundation.

COMMON MISALIGNMENTS

- Weight uneven from front to back, position too short
- Hands or elbows rolling outward
- Shoulders pinched
- Ribs/abdomen collapsed
- Back rounded from tight shoulders, hamstrings or both

ASSISTS

For uneven weight: Down Dog should look like a nice inverted "V" shape, weight distributed equally between hands and feet. Start by setting hand/foot pattern: hands shoulder-width and feet hip-width apart. Spacing on mat is also important. Beginners and advanced students tend to walk in their Dog, shortening space between hands and feet. When they come forward into Plank, the feet and hands have to re-adjust. Instead, lengthen the space in between, so that the average student covers about seventy to eighty percent of their mat, measured from hands to feet, maintaining that spacing throughout Surya Namaskar. Heels are slightly off floor, so legs stay active. These small adjustments help students settle into better position and proportion, relative to the floor.

For hand/elbow alignment: In Down Dog, solid hand-to-floor contact is essential to transmit strength up through wrists, forearms and upper arms to the shoulders. If you see the hands rolling outward (among muscular men/beginning women students, usually), reset them slightly further apart, *firmly* pressing down on both hands to reinforce good connection to floor. For wrist pain, try rolling up front of mat to gently elevate the base or "heel" of hands so that upper palms and fingers are slightly lower than the wrists; use roll for Down Dog, Plank and Chaturanga. For elbows rolling out, take hold of upper arms, firmly rotating outer, upper arms outward and *away* from ears (elbow creases spin to face each other, or slightly forward toward front of mat). If Down Dog is held for several breaths, place a block in between the forearms to help realign the lower arms or correct hyper-extension of elbows.

To align shoulders: Pinching or hanging into the shoulders is far and away the most universal misalignment in Down Dog. When this happens, the shoulders get "stuck" and lose their ability to conduct energy and strength from the hands to the feet. The upper arm roll, described above, helps bring shoulders onto the back and away from neck/ears. Your touch might be subtle or quite firm—especially when assisting men. You may have to repeat the assist many times before the arms learn to realign. You might also massage and then hug the trapezius muscles down the back, to help to bring shoulders into better alignment.

Extra Love: The Art of Hands-on Assists

For collapsed ribs/abdomen: Common for flexible, advanced students, the back will hyper-extend, pushing ribs forward and compressing the shoulders. Hyper-extension is visible from above (yoga top scrunches at back body) or from the side (ribs/front body hang down toward mat). Terrifically stretchy as it may feel, hyper-extended alignment eventually stresses the shoulders or lower back, the habit becoming so ingrained that students have trouble self-adjusting in Down Dog and other poses. Point out the hyper-extension to students, then, to assist, put one hand flat under ribs and help to draw them into front body. There should be no arch in lower back. Side waists remain long, lower abdomen drawing up (*uddiyana bandha*). Reinforce this assist regularly.

For rounded back/tight hamstrings: Start by resetting the foot pattern, allowing a little extra length between hands/feet. Have student bend knees slightly, keeping sit bones lifted, *as* they press hands firmly into floor and try to lengthen spine. Press or slide one hand down the back toward sacrum to suggest length. Aim for full extension without tension/gripping.

Other great assists for added extension/stretch: Sacrum press: lunging in front, press sacrum back and up with both hands, aiming to bring more traction into spine and length to back body. Your press is *firm*, moving energy back and at a slight diagonal up, in line with spine. Hip pull: standing behind, firmly hold around front thigh crease and pull hips up and back toward you, drawing spine long, anchoring strength into student's legs. Thigh pull: cross your wrists between their legs and hold inner thighs from the front to pull straight back, giving legs a slight inner spiral along with the tug. These assists are best for intermediate/advanced students with good alignment and some flexibility or "give" in the pose. They must always come from a strong foundation first.

Surya Namaskar continues with a step, lunge or jump forward into Flat Back or Uttanasana, followed by Urdhva Hastasana and finishing with Tadasana. You might repeat and reinforce the same assists you did for these poses at the beginning of the sequence, or try new ones.

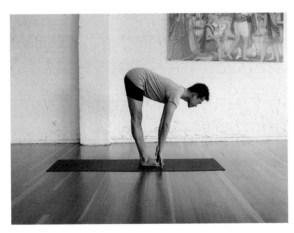
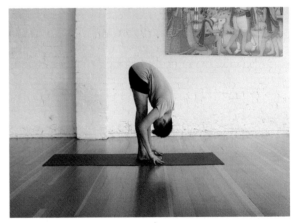
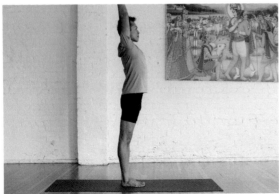
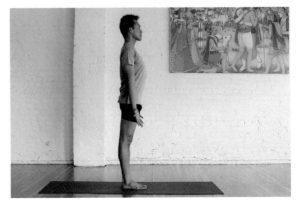

ASSISTING VARIATIONS FOR SURYA NAMASKAR

This section shows several different assisting variations for Surya Namaskar. Here is where you would "mix and match" different assists depending on the overall effect — lighter touch, grounding, deepening, etc.,— you'd like to deliver, in addition to the level of student. The previous section familiarized you with assisting/ adjusting options for each of the poses. Now that you're familiar with a vocabulary of different assists, you can study and practice these variations. Each variation has a short description, indicated assists and thumbnail photos as a guide.

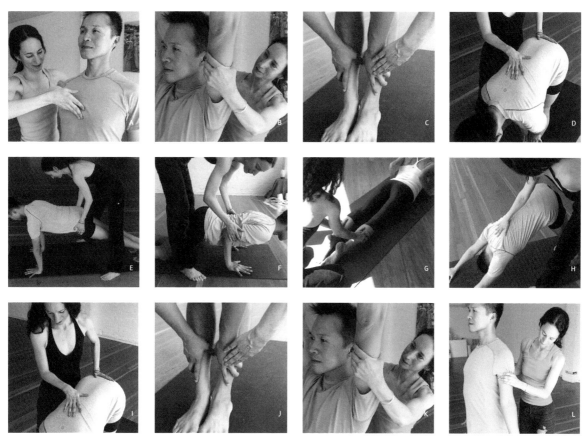

VARIATION 1 - MODIFIED/BEGINNERS: LIGHT

Appropriate for new/beginning students, with a lighter touch on the assists
(a) Tadasana - sternum lift; (b) Urdhva Hastasana - align arms; (c) Uttanasana — position hands on shins; (d) Prepare/Flat Back - hands/shins; (e) Plank - hold hips; (f) Modified/Half Chaturanga — support elbows as knees lower; (g) Bhujangasana - anchor feet/calves; (h) Adho Mukha Svanasana — lightly slide hand down back; (i) Step Forward to Flat Back — position hands on shins; (j) Uttanasana — hands on shins; (k) Urdhva Hastasana - align arms; (l) Tadasana — lightly rotate upper arms

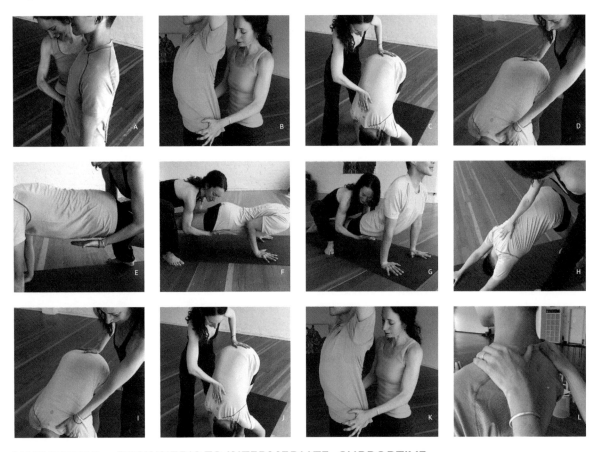

VARIATION 2 – BEGINNER'S TO INTERMEDIATE: SUPPORTIVE

More supportive assists, slightly firmer touch, for students gaining familiarity with the sequence
(a) Tadasana – anchor sacrum/abdomen lift; (b) Urdhva Hastasana – hip hug; (c) Uttanasana – sacrum/back press; (d) Prepare/Flat Back – sacrum press/support shoulder; (e) Plank – Spatula; (f) Chaturanga – Forklift (or hold thighs); (g) Urdhva Mukha Svanasana – Forklift; (h) Adho Mukha Svanasana – hand slide down back; (i) Jump/Step Forward to Flat Back – sacrum press/support shoulder; (j) Uttanasana – sacrum/back press; (k) Urdhva Hastasana – hip hug; (l) Tadasana – press trapezius down

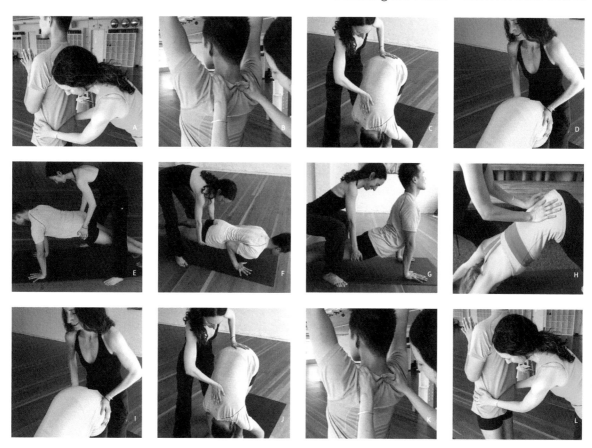

VARIATION 3: INTERMEDIATE TO ADVANCED: GROUNDING

Intermediate to Advanced students, with assists and adjustments to give a firm sense of grounding
(a) Tadasana – firm hip hug; (b) Urdhva Hastasana – firm trapezius press; (c) Uttanasana – sacrum/back press; (d) Prepare/Flat Back – Seat Squeeze; (e) Plank – hold hips; (f) Chaturanga – hold thighs; (g) Urdhva Mukha Svanasana – hold thighs; (h) Adho Mukha Svanasana – come around to front for sacrum press; (i) Jump/Step Forward to Flat Back – Seat Squeeze; (j) Uttanasana – sacrum/back press; (k) Urdhva Hastasana – trapezius press; (l) Tadasana – firm hip hug

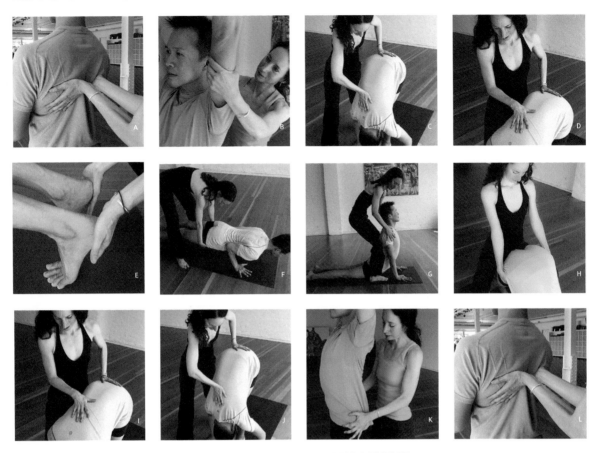

VARIATION 4 – INTERMEDIATE TO ADVANCED: EXPANSIVE

Intermediate to Advanced students, these assists are lengthening and expansive

(a) Tadasana – lift back ribs; (b) Urdhva Hastasana – rotate arms; (c) Uttanasana – sacrum/back press; (d) Prepare/Flat Back – sacrum press/hand slide; (e) Plank – press heels; (f) Chaturanga – step in and hold hips; (g) Urdhva Mukha Svanasana – knees to back; (h) Adho Mukha Svanasana – thigh pull; (i) Jump/Step Forward to Flat Back – sacrum press/hand slide; (j) Uttanasana – sacrum/back press; (k) Urdhva Hastasana – hip hug; (l) Tadasana – lift back ribs

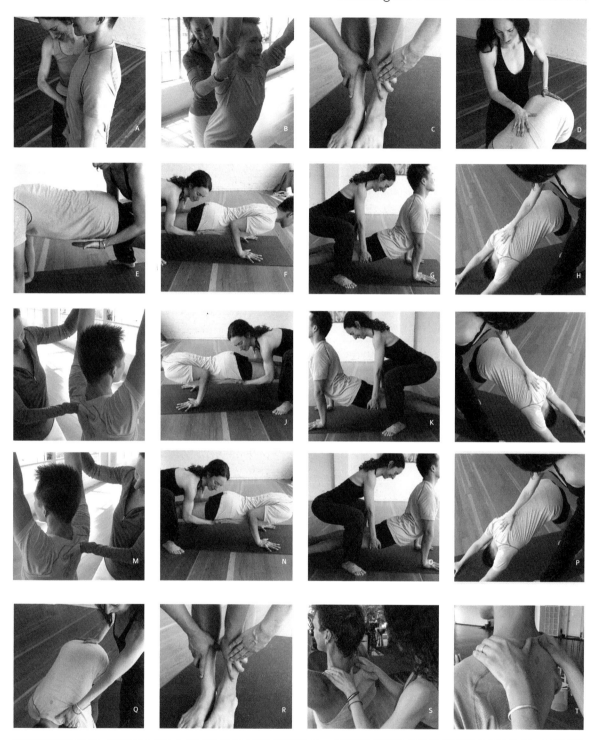

VARIATION 5: ASHTANGA SUN SALUTATION B – BEGINNER TO INTERMEDIATE: LIGHT

Offering lighter assists/refinements to the classic B series Sun Salutation

(a) Tadasana - sacrum/abdomen assist; (b) Utkatasana – rotate upper arms; (c) Uttanasana –position hands on shins; (d) Prepare/Flat Back – sacrum press/hand slide; (e) Plank – Spatula; (f) Chaturanga – Forklift; (g) Urdhva Mukha Svanasana – hold thighs; (h) Adho Mukha Svanasana – slide hand lightly down back; (i) Virabhadrasana 1, Right Side - support back of heart, extending arms up; (j) Chaturanga – Forklift; (k) Urdhva Mukha Svanasana – hold thighs;

(l) Adho Mukha Svanasana – slide hand down back; (m) Virabhadrasana 1, Left Side - support back of heart, help extend arms up; (n) Chaturanga – Forkift ; (o) Urdhva Mukha Svanasana – hold thighs; (p) Adho Mukha Svanasana – slide hand down back; (q) Prepare/Flat Back – sacrum press/support shoulder; (r) Uttanasana – position hands on shins; (s) Utkatasana – lightly press trapezius down; (t) Tadasana – lightly press trapezius down

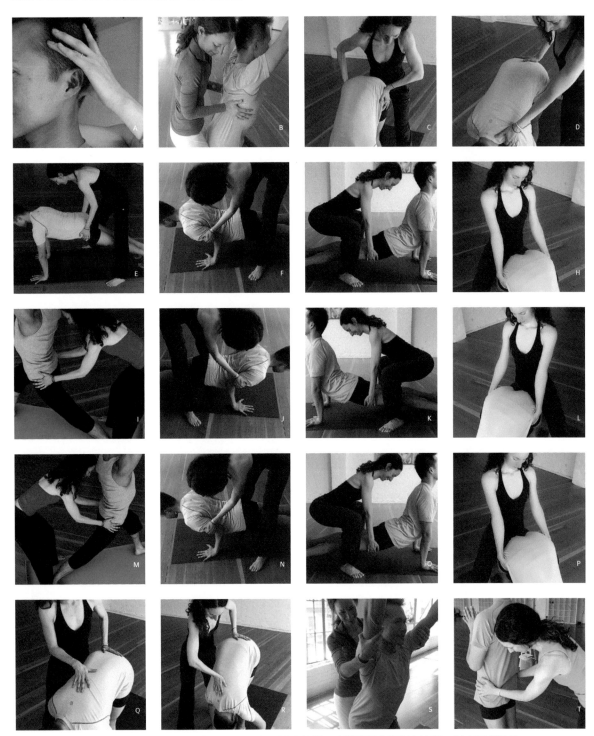

VARIATION 6: ASHTANGA SUN SALUTATION B - INTERMEDIATE: ALIGNING

Focusing on precise alignment and form, for Intermediate students

(a) Tadasana - lengthen neck/fingers around head; (b) Utkatasana – anchor hips, align torso; (c) Uttanasana – Seat Squeeze/align hips; (d) Prepare/Flat Back – sacrum press/shoulder support; (e) Plank –hold hips; (f) Chaturanga – wrist/elbow alignment; (g) Urdhva Mukha Svanasana – hold thighs; (h) Adho Mukha Svanasana – thigh pull; (i) Virabhadrasana 1, Right Side – anchor back foot/square hips; (j) Chaturanga – wrist/elbow alignment; (k) Urdhva Mukha Svanasana – hold thighs; (l) Adho Mukha Svanasana – thigh pull; (m) Virabhadrasana 1, Left Side – anchor back foot/square hips; (n) Chaturanga –wrist/elbow alignment; (o) Urdhva Mukha Svanasana – hold hips; (p) Adho Mukha Svanasana – thigh pull; (q) Prepare/Flat Back – sacrum press/hand slide; (r) Uttanasana – sacrum/back press; (s) Utkatasana – rotate/align arms; (t) Tadasana – hip hug

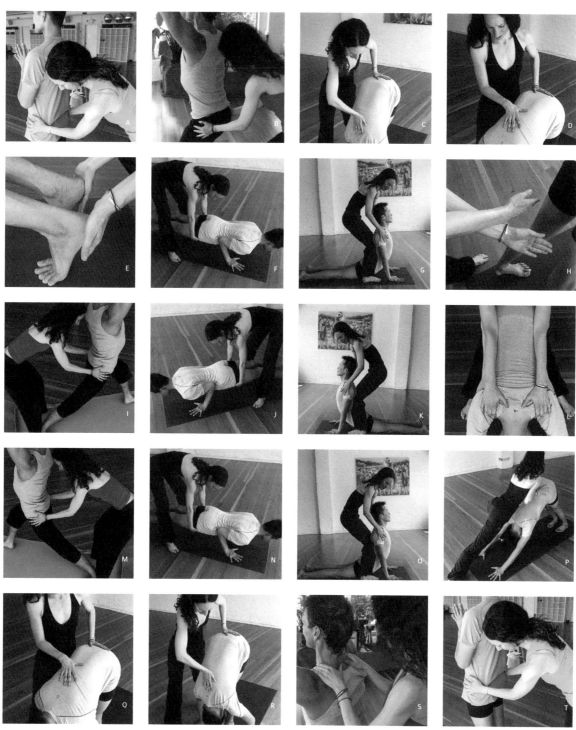

VARIATION 7: ASHTANGA SUN SALUTATION B – INTERMEDIATE TO ADVANCED: DEEPENING
Deeper assists and adjustments for students with strong alignment

(a) Tadasana – hip hug; (b) Utkatasana – Seat Squeeze (firm touch, encourage deeper bend in knees); (c) Uttanasana – sacrum/back press; (d) Prepare/Flat Back – sacrum press/hand slide; (e) Plank – step behind and press heels; (f) Chaturanga – hold hips; (g) Urdhva Mukha Svanasana – knees to back; (h) Adho Mukha Svanasana – cross wrist/ firm thigh pull; (i) Virabhadrasana 1, Right Side – anchor back foot/square hips, or deepen lunge in front leg; (j) Chaturanga – hold hips; (k) Urdhva Mukha Svanasana – knees to back; (l) Adho Mukha Svanasana – firmly pull trapezius/shoulders back; (m) Virabhadrasana 1, Left Side – anchor back foot/square hips, or deepen lunge in front leg; (n) Chaturanga – hold hips; (o) Urdhva Mukha Svanasana – knees to back; (p) Adho Mukha Svanasana – firm sacrum press; (q) Prepare/Flat Back – sacrum press/hand slide; (r) Uttanasana – sacrum/firm back press; (s) Utkatasana – press trapezius firmly down; (t) Tadasana – firm hip hug

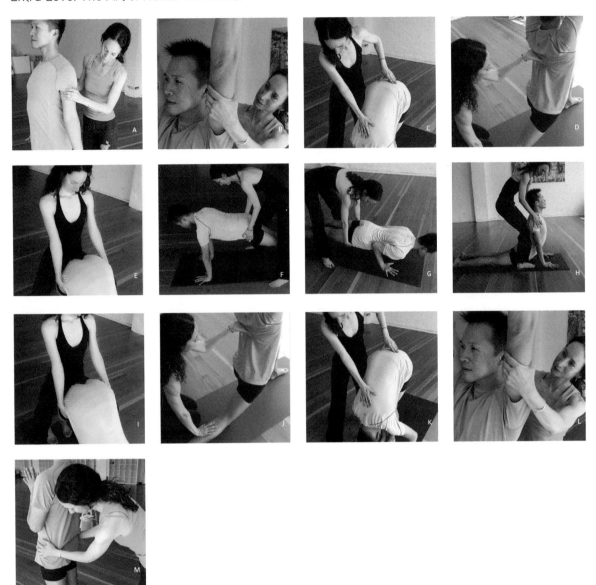

VARIATION 8: SUN SALUTATION WITH LOW LUNGE – ALL LEVELS: MODERATE

Moderate intensity assists, incorporating assisting for Low Lunge

(a) Tadasana – roll arms open; (b) Urdhva Hastasana – rotate arms; (c) Uttanasana – sacrum/back press;
(d) Low Lunge - anchor calf/support back of heart; (e) Adho Mukha Svanasana – thigh pull; (f) Plank – hold
thighs; (g) Chaturanga – hold hips; (h) Urdhva Mukha Svanasana – knees to back; (i) Adho Mukha Svanasana
– thigh pull; (j) Low Lunge – anchor calf/support back of heart; (k) Uttanasana – sacrum/back press; (l) Urdhva
Hastasana – rotate arms; (m) Tadasana – hip hug

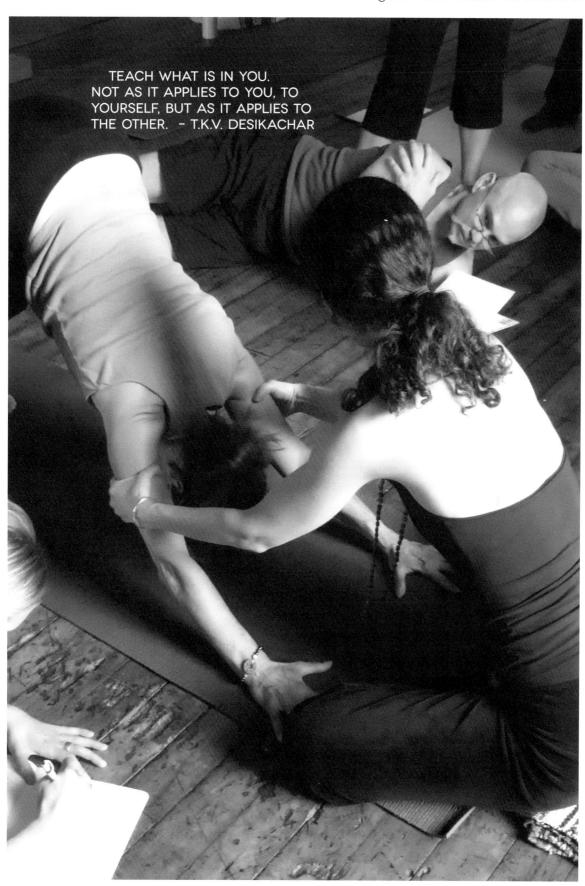

TEACH WHAT IS IN YOU.
NOT AS IT APPLIES TO YOU, TO
YOURSELF, BUT AS IT APPLIES TO
THE OTHER. - T.K.V. DESIKACHAR

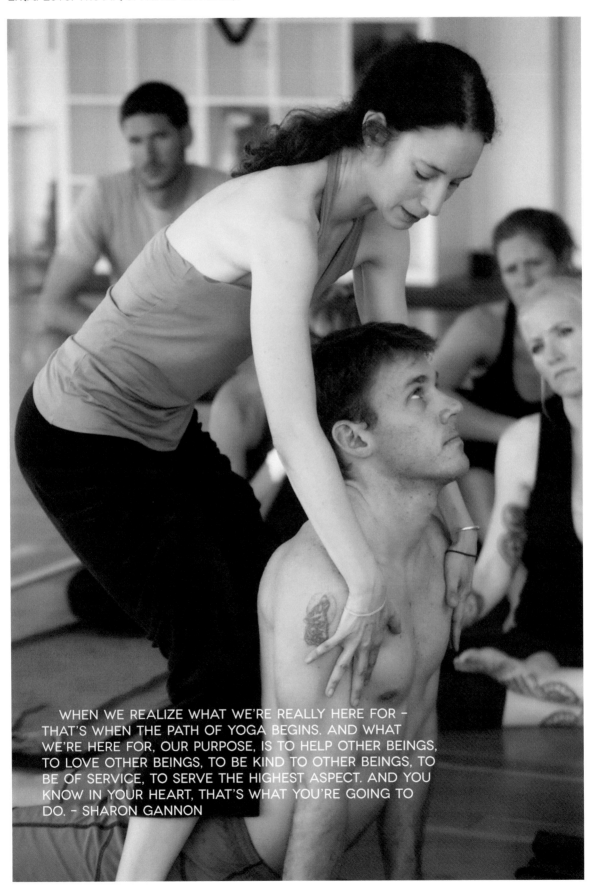

WHEN WE REALIZE WHAT WE'RE REALLY HERE FOR –
THAT'S WHEN THE PATH OF YOGA BEGINS. AND WHAT
WE'RE HERE FOR, OUR PURPOSE, IS TO HELP OTHER BEINGS,
TO LOVE OTHER BEINGS, TO BE KIND TO OTHER BEINGS, TO
BE OF SERVICE, TO SERVE THE HIGHEST ASPECT. AND YOU
KNOW IN YOUR HEART, THAT'S WHAT YOU'RE GOING TO
DO. – SHARON GANNON

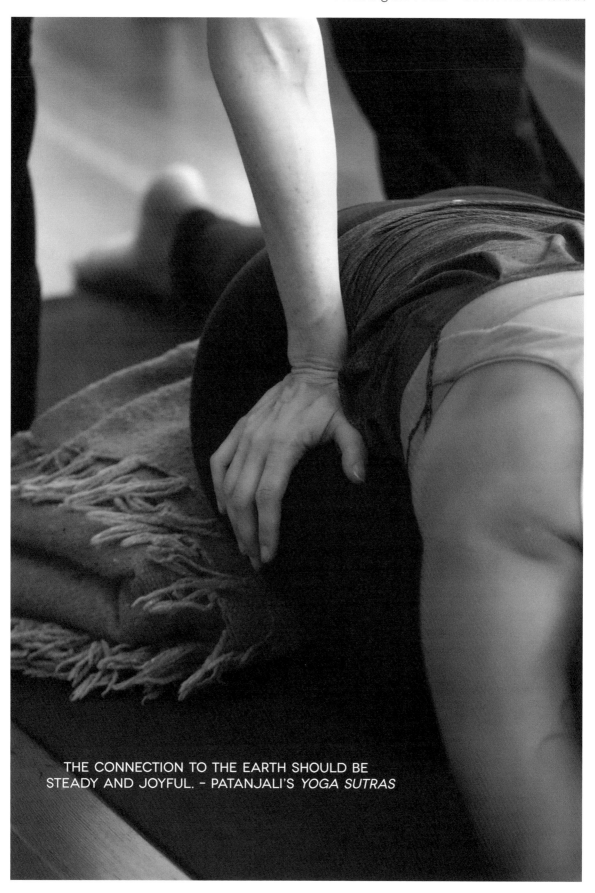

THE CONNECTION TO THE EARTH SHOULD BE
STEADY AND JOYFUL. – PATANJALI'S *YOGA SUTRAS*

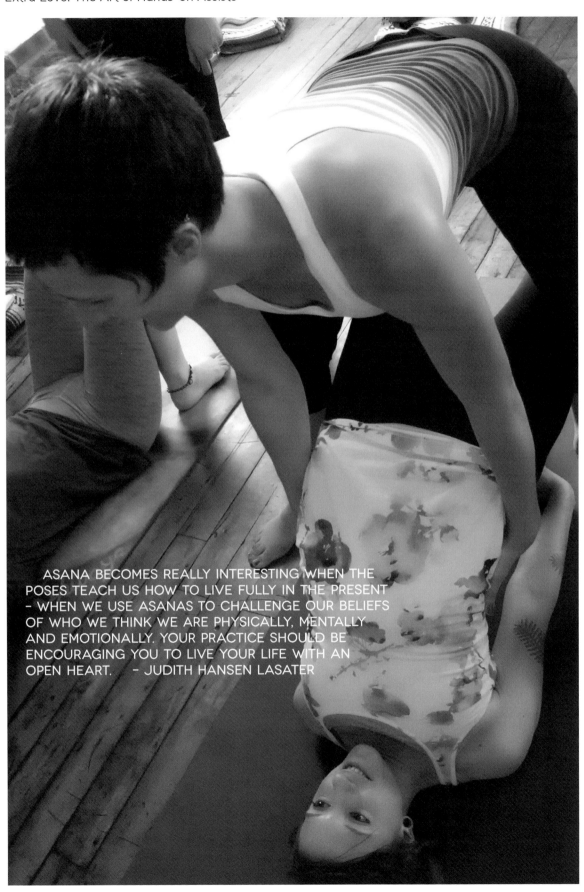

ASANA BECOMES REALLY INTERESTING WHEN THE POSES TEACH US HOW TO LIVE FULLY IN THE PRESENT - WHEN WE USE ASANAS TO CHALLENGE OUR BELIEFS OF WHO WE THINK WE ARE PHYSICALLY, MENTALLY AND EMOTIONALLY. YOUR PRACTICE SHOULD BE ENCOURAGING YOU TO LIVE YOUR LIFE WITH AN OPEN HEART.   - JUDITH HANSEN LASATER

ETHICS/SAFETY CONSIDERATIONS

Your best foundation for ethics and safety considerations is found under "Principles of Hands-on Assists." I mentioned there and it bears repeating, that a student's experience at all levels is YOUR responsibility. Do not attempt an assist unless you have 100% confidence. Practice with a few poses, perfect your technique, then move on to others. I also said that you need to protect yourself as well, using proper breath and *mula bandha* (root lock) while assisting, proper technique and stance, carry liability insurance – which is required at all if not most studios and follow professional teaching guidelines. Most schools include these guidelines as part of teacher training. The Yoga Alliance has a general code of conduct on their website (www.yogaalliance.org).

What the professional guidelines may not go into are the subtle nuances inherent in assisting. From the student's side, you may be rejected, told you are wrong, or told that the student doesn't do the pose "that way." You may receive an unspoken, emotional download from a student, expressed as stress, tension, aggression, sadness or other emotions. A student may also transmit emotional neediness, or a flat-out sexual "charge." A very pretty friend of mine has a (male) student who grabs her wrist and lets out a loud moan, any time she assists him in Triangle Pose. Recognize that people bring their stories/needs into the classroom and may unconsciously look to you for resolution.

A STUDENT'S EXPERIENCE AT ALL LEVELS IS YOUR RESPONSIBILITY.
DO NOT ATTEMPT AN ASSIST UNLESS YOU HAVE 100% CONFIDENCE.

To get yourself into the mindset of assisting with utmost professionalism, I tell teachers to embody – to the letter – *brahmacharya*. From the Yoga Sutras, *brahmacharya* is commonly translated as celibacy or sexual continence. Practically speaking, it means personal energy management. You draw a very careful boundary around your energetic field, so as to neither project nor make yourself receptive to any sexual or sensual charge *whatsoever.* In other words, you do not merge your energy with that of the student. The boundary is apparent from your manner, professionalism and technique.

Extra Love: The Art of Hands-on Assists

Today's Yoga studios are still outlets for students' self expression, creativity, athleticism, femininity, machismo, sensuality and even exhibitionism. So I cannot say enough about knowing, following and projecting proper ethical guidelines.

When you teach or assist, dress professionally. Do not wear dangly jewelry, clunky rings or bracelets. Keep your nails trim. Carry a small hand towel(s) and use it to avoid passing sweat from one student to another, or to keep your own perspiration in check. I am not shy about asking men to keep their shirts on, or switch to a dry tank top, so that I can assist them more effectively. If you are working in a heated room, where everyone is very sweaty, lay a towel down as a buffer between your hands or body and your contact point with the student. The towel gives you better traction for your assist, helps absorb extra sweat and creates a protective layer honoring the student's physical space.

Finally, a word about injuries and pregnancy, which we cover more in-depth in my workshops. Usually a student with an injury or who is pregnant will let you know before class. In San Francisco, a few studios have poker chips or small cards students put on their mats, indicating "hands off!" Some teachers also check in with students at the beginning, or invite students to opt out of hands-on assists if they prefer. Teachers might say, "I am going to be assisting during class – if you do not want to be touched, please let me know." I assume that a student is open to hands-on assists unless she tells me otherwise. If I'm not sure, I ask. Strive to cultivate openness and trust, so that students feel safe telling you what they need and to ensure you feel no awkwardness or hesitation about assisting students with special needs. Know the contraindications for injuries, expecting moms and other special needs and advise students about how to modify.

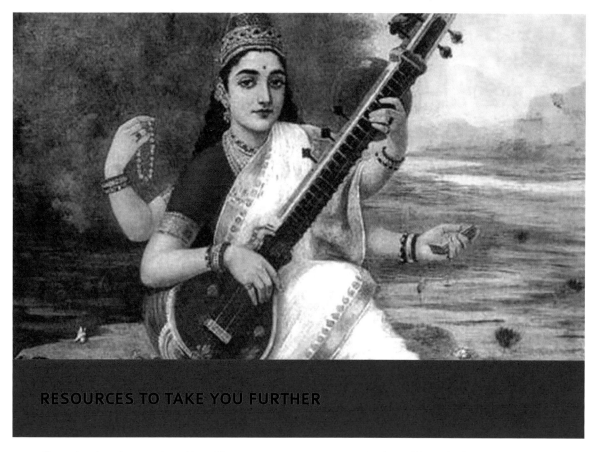

RESOURCES TO TAKE YOU FURTHER

Since the time I started my Yoga library twenty years ago, we've been blessed with an avalanche of new resources for Yoga teachers, to accompany the old standbys. These favorite books illuminate the art of alignment and/or the development and inner essence of Yoga poses, in crystal clear and insightful ways. I recommend these books to teachers who want in-depth information to serve their assisting skills.

Yoga the Iyengar Way, by Silva Mehta — A beautifully illustrated book with focus on precision and alignment.

Light on Yoga, by B.K.S. Iyengar — The all-time classic.

Yoga Anatomy, by Leslie Kaminoff — Anatomy presented in-depth, including anatomy of the breath.

Jivamukti Yoga: Practices for Liberating Body & Spirit, by Sharon Gannon and David Life — By my teachers, a life-changing book for yogis of all stripes. Chapters on Prana, Asana and Vinyasa Krama are especially relevant for hands-on assisting.

Yoga Body: The Origins of Modern Posture Practice, by Mark Singleton — A fascinating history of how modern yoga poses originated and developed into the modern era.

Hatha Yoga Pradipika, by Yogi Swatmarama — The classic (before Iyengar's *Light on Yoga*), a must-read for serious teachers. I like the Bihar School of Yoga edition.

The Tibetan Book of Yoga: Ancient Buddhist Teachings on the Philosophy and Practice of Yoga, by Geshe Michael Roach — The Tibetan Heart Yoga lineage offers exquisite reflections on the subtle body and inner form.

Eastern Body, Western Mind: Psychology and the Chakra System as a Path to the Self, by Anodea Judith — A practical, in-depth examination of the chakra system that will take your teaching and assisting insights to the next level.

Anatomy of the Spirit: The Seven Stages of Power and Healing, by Caroline Myss — Useful insights you can apply to student evaluation, healing and empowerment, from a master energy healer. Intuition, she believes, is not a gift but an acquired skill.

American Yoga: The Paths and Practices of America's Greatest Yoga Masters, by Carrie Schneider and Andy Ryan — A beautiful, coffee table book, with personal stories and approaches to asana.

The Tree of Yoga, by B.K.S. Iyengar — Reflections about Yoga and the cycle of life, in this little gem of a book.

Meditations from the Mat: Daily Reflections on the Path of Yoga, by Rolf Gates — An intimate journey into Yoga's key themes, starting with the Yoga Sutras.

ABOUT THE AUTHOR

JILL ABELSON

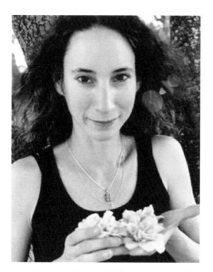

Jill Abelson is a bi-coastal Yoga instructor, teacher trainer, workshop presenter and one of the Yoga world's leading educators in the art of hands-on assists. Yoga Alliance registered (E-RYT500), her extensive training includes Jivamukti, Ashtanga, Vinyasa and Kripalu Yoga. In 2007, she was recognized by Yoga Journal as one of the "Five Yogis Changing the World." Her unique and uncanny sense of the human body draws from a lifetime of dance, athletics and Yoga. Volume One of Jill's *Extra Love: The Art of Hands-on Assists* has won wide praise for weaving knowledge learned from master teachers of various styles of yoga to produce an "essential tool for teachers, assistants and yoga teaching trainees." She presents her popular assists workshops and training sessions at studios across the country.

www.yogaofliberation.com

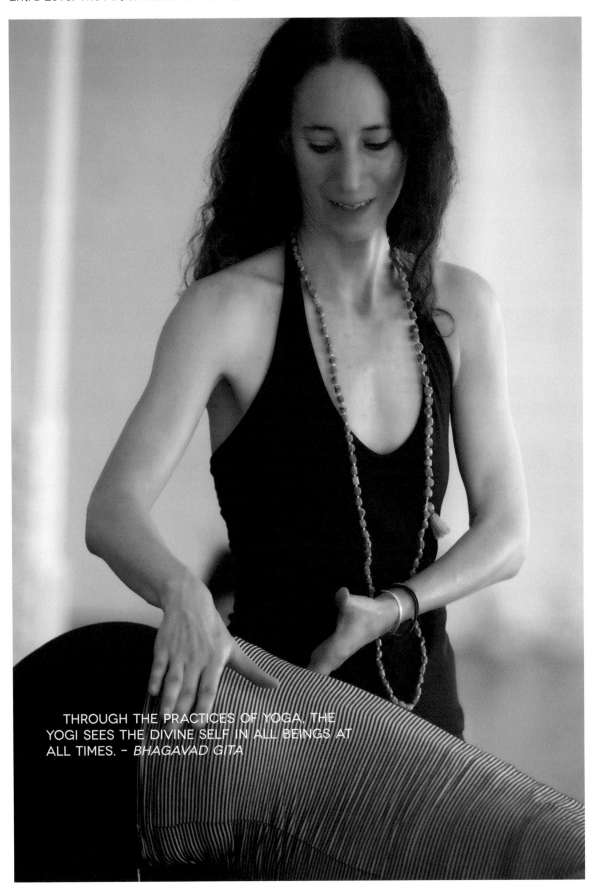

THROUGH THE PRACTICES OF YOGA, THE YOGI SEES THE DIVINE SELF IN ALL BEINGS AT ALL TIMES. - *BHAGAVAD GITA*

ACKOWLEDGEMENTS

First and foremost, profound thanks and appreciation to Michael Fantasia, my designer and patient guide, who brought the first and second Manuals to light and to Tom Lee, dear friend and dedicated San Francisco Yoga teacher, who beautifully modeled the majority of poses in Volume 1 and again here. With their open hearts, Jennifer Jarrett and Joseph Melone graced the section on Back Bends and Standing Poses.

For hosting the events and workshops pictured here and for creating incredible communities for learning and growth, deep thanks go to Project Yoga Richmond, in Richmond, VA; Flow Yoga Center in Washington, DC; Carrboro Yoga Company in Carrboro, NC; Integral Yoga Institute in New York City; Yoga Tree in San Francisco, CA; and Urban Flow, also in San Francisco, CA, who generously provided studio space for our photo shoots.

To the students, friends and teachers pictured in the Manual, including Elizabeth Rosser, Katie Raycroft, Niav Connor, Sarah McTee, Agatha Glowacki, Tarek Ghany, Adam Lapierre, Courtney Long, Fran Morfesis, Victoria Bowden and Natasha Zaslove, thank you for the opportunity to continue inspiring one another.

Contributing photographers include Michael Fantasia, Richard Jenrette, Rob Kunkle and Ximena Guttierez.

My copy editor, Joslyn Hamilton, provided an expert outside eye and invaluable support.

Once again to Ben Lorica and Alon Sagee, thank you for encouraging me to put my knowledge onto paper.

And to Jeff, all my love.

For information on workshops or teacher trainings, please visit www.yogaofliberation.com.

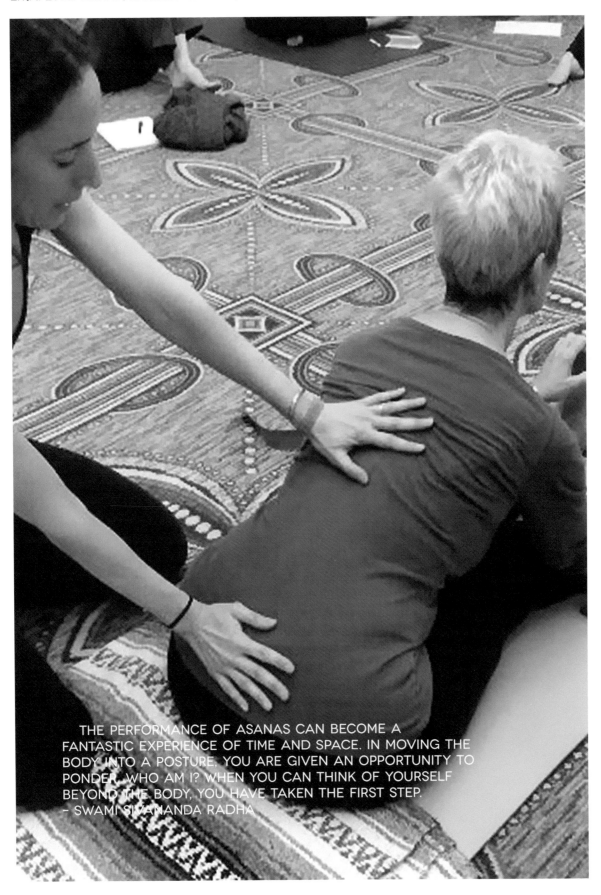

THE PERFORMANCE OF ASANAS CAN BECOME A
FANTASTIC EXPERIENCE OF TIME AND SPACE. IN MOVING THE
BODY INTO A POSTURE, YOU ARE GIVEN AN OPPORTUNITY TO
PONDER, WHO AM I? WHEN YOU CAN THINK OF YOURSELF
BEYOND THE BODY, YOU HAVE TAKEN THE FIRST STEP.
– SWAMI SIVANANDA RADHA

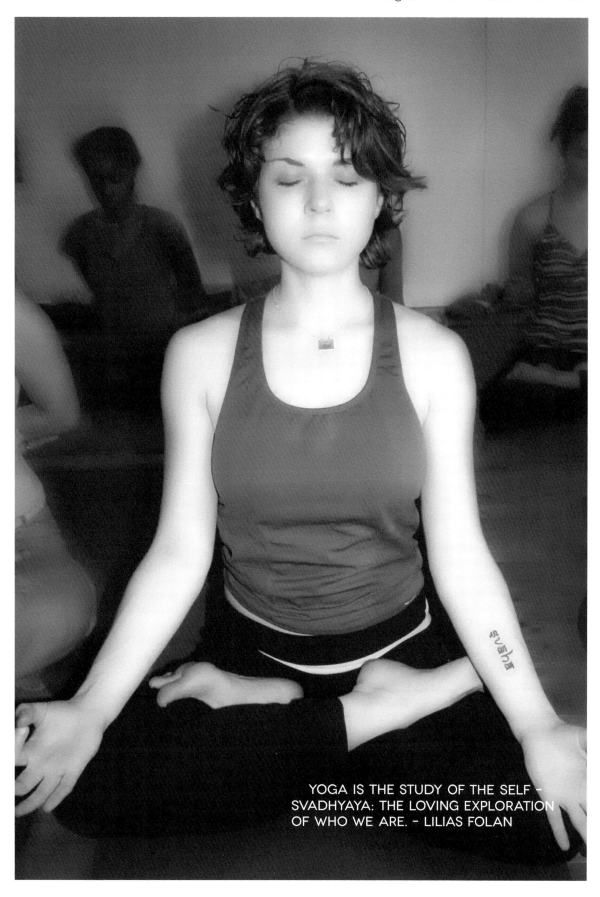

YOGA IS THE STUDY OF THE SELF -
SVADHYAYA: THE LOVING EXPLORATION
OF WHO WE ARE. - LILIAS FOLAN

CPSIA information can be obtained
at www.ICGtesting.com
Printed in the USA
LVIC06n1506310114
371837LV00013B/108